"You are not the brightest of my four sons"

...and other depressing things that have been said to me.

How I use humor and reframing in my struggles with mental illness, its stigma, and words that hurt.

John Shuchart

with James Blasingame and Marianne Wasson

"You are not the brightest of my four sons"
…and other depressing things that have been said to me.

How I use humor and reframing in my struggles with mental illness, its stigma, and words that hurt.
By John Shuchart with Marianne Wasson and James Blasingame

Copyright © 2015 John Shuchart. All rights reserved.

Published by
The Shuchart Group, LLC.
P.O. Box 651
Collinsville, IL 62234
www.notthebrightest.com

ISBN: 978-0-9908555-0-7

For further information, contact the publisher.

Cover design by Jim Fortune
Caricature by Steve Nyman
Interior design by Nick Zelinger

First Edition

Printed by MEDiAHEAD! in the United States of America

For my wife, Stevie

For everyone living with a mental illness

*For all of those working to help eliminate the
stigma associated with the disease*

A Very Special Tribute

My wife's Aunt, Liz Bohm, could *never* have written this book. You see, most everyone you and I have ever met (me especially) gets angry at times. We hold grudges; we say negative things about people. We have bad days where we feel glum and think the world isn't quite as rosy as we'd like it to be.

Aunt Liz is different. The world is *always* rosy. Every day is a *wonderful* day. People are to be loved, honored and respected, not criticized and held in contempt. Anger only hurts you, not others, so forgive and forget quickly and find that which is good in absolutely everyone. Smile…often. It will brighten your day and others', too.

Now approaching her 90th year on this earth, Aunt Liz has been a gift to everyone who has had the privilege of knowing her, but no one could have benefited more than me. You see, it's impossible not to be like her when you're in her presence. You can't frown, and you can't complain about others. You find yourself reacting to her glow, her warmth and you, too think, "today is a wonderful day." It's impossible to be depressed in Aunt Liz's company.

Two people Aunt Liz has certainly touched are Stewart and Esther Stein. As Stewart is a former law partner of Aunt Liz's husband, he and his wife have known Liz for over 35 years and have been selfless in their nurturing and caring for her, especially as she has become a widow and begun to age. But, their love and attention to Liz is not a surprise: both Stewart and Esther are committed people who spend an inordinate amount of their time, energy, and money working to better the entire Kansas City community. The Steins are exactly the kind of people Aunt Liz appreciates: loving, caring, and always knowing that today will be a special day.

Table of Contents

Foreword

Dear Friends,

Mental illnesses are pervasive. Few if any of us can claim that there is no one in our extended family or circle of friends and colleagues who is not affected. We know that the majority of children and adults who experience mental illness are not in treatment and that the cost of untreated mental illness represents a huge human and financial toll in the billions of dollars per year. Stigma associated with mental illness is a primary barrier to addressing these issues.

NAMI believes in the value of treatment and recovery from mental illness. For many, this process begins with acknowledging their symptoms and taking charge of the recovery process. John Shuchart's witty stories captured in this book reflect his own struggles and willingness to move on with his life even in the face of many challenges. It's a testimony to overcoming mental illness and to challenging the stigma that has been so widely associated with these disorders. I trust that you will find John's stories inspiring in the way that he has been able to re-frame experiences that life has dealt him.

We are committed to working with John and many others to communicate positive messages about mental health recovery. We invite you to connect with NAMI in your local community and to get involved with our programs of peer support, education and advocacy. As the largest grass-roots mental health advocacy organization in the U.S., we have programs available to educate those affected by mental illness, their family members, and the community at-large.

Enjoy this funny, poignant book and join the fight to reduce mental health stigma.

Rick Cagan
Executive Director

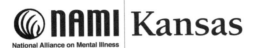

Preface

"You are not the brightest of my four sons"

"Everything is funny, as long as it's happening to somebody else."
—Will Rogers

A few years ago, I told my wife, Stevie, that one of these days I was going to write a book. She asked me what it would be about, and I told her that I wasn't sure, but that it would have something to do with my living with depression. She told me I was crazy.

In Stevie's defense, she was basing her opinion on facts: over the past dozen years I've been to psychiatrists, psychologists, and various other therapists in seeking treatment for depression. I even spent ten days in a leading psychiatric hospital. I have to admit that many days have been extremely dark and scary, and there have been more than a few times I've considered taking my own life. On one particular occasion, I came frighteningly close.

It occurred a few years after I was T-boned by a distracted driver. He ran a red light, smashing my car to bits, and although I was uninjured at first, over the next ten years I needed more than fifteen orthopedic operations to keep my body together. During that time I became frustrated with all of the poking and prodding, the years of painful physical therapy, and the false confidences espoused by my doctors about their abilities to improve my condition. I took opiates for the many hours of pain I endured, and after years of popping those magical little pills, I became addicted. To me, my future was hopeless; one operation would simply lead to another, to be followed by yet several more. My mood soured and turned into one of deep depression, leading me to plan my suicide.

In arranging a suicide, there are a couple of important, somewhat obvious decisions that have to be made, such as *how* and *where* to do it. And I guess a third decision would be *when*, but that's easier to decide once you've got answers to the first two. In my case, the "how" was particularly important: it had to be done as quickly and as painlessly as possible (I'm basically a wimp). It would also have to happen late in the day so I'd have time for a final trip to Dairy Queen for a medium – or, why not a *large*? – Blizzard, with pecans.

In order to determine the most painless way out, I spent a couple of hours surfing the Internet and eventually made the decision to use carbon monoxide poisoning. I read that all I had to do was turn my car engine on, and be in an enclosed space where the gas couldn't escape. The Internet said if I rolled down my windows and remembered to fill the gas tank (you wouldn't believe how many people try to do this with the needle near empty!) that the whole process wouldn't take very long and would *probably* be 100 percent painless.

All that was left was for me to find a place where I could park my car and not be discovered until it was over. I certainly didn't want Stevie to have to go through the trauma of discovering my body, so using my own garage wasn't an option. I thought about borrowing a friend's – or using the garage of someone who owed me money – but I decided that was too morbid. As I mulled my options, I drove to my pharmacy to renew one of my antidepressant medications. *Why* I thought I needed to renew it when I was going to be dead soon is beyond me, but on the way there, I got lost; after all, I had a few other things on my mind. As I began to turn my car around and head back to pick up my prescription, I noticed a rental storage facility – the kind where each unit is built like its own individual garage. Right away I was thinking, "That's perfect. I just need to drive my car into the unit, pull down the door, turn on my engine, and finish my Blizzard."

Later, I went online to get the name and exact address of the facility. During my search, results for several other garage-type storage units popped up, including one that was closer to my home than the one I had seen. I clicked on the website and saw that they were running a special: *Sign a two-year contract and get the first month's rent, free!* A month's rent, *free*, and all I had to be willing to do was to sign a two-year agreement? Heck, I'd be willing to sign a ten-year agreement, or even a lifetime one! Why would I care? This was great!

And then, something very unexpected happened: I began laughing and I couldn't stop! I'm thinking, "Here I am about to kill myself, and I'm concerned about the freaking cost, and excited about getting a 'deal'!" As I was laughing, I noticed that my sadness was starting to recede. In fact, my entire mood was shifting, becoming elevated to a level I hadn't experienced in a long, long time. Wow! I liked this feeling! Dying…I never really wanted to die (does anyone, really?); I just wanted to feel like *this*!

Researchers have known for a while now what I had discovered by accident: that our bodies have *endorphins*, chemicals that have the ability to act like a kind of morphine for us. They're always present, but they need to be released, and although there are several ways to do that, *one of the most effective is through laughing!*

As much as I appreciated my new mood, I didn't relish the idea of maintaining it by spending the rest of my life thinking of funny ways to do myself in! While I understood that laughter had saved me, I knew my challenge would be learning to think of humorous things as often as I could, since doing so would keep me from falling back into what I call the Dark Hole of Depression. But, since I'm not a comedian and can't remember even the shortest and funniest of jokes, I needed an effective tool to help me find things to laugh about. Fortunately, I remembered something one of my therapists taught me. She'd once asked me to recall the earliest traumatic event in my life. She wanted me to revisit the event and "reframe" it. She said that, just like when we change a frame on a painting and it often times alters the way it appears, I could change the way an event looked to me by changing its frame. She wasn't suggesting that I could change what had happened (she was good…but not *that* good), but I could change my *perception* of it. The result would be that this earliest traumatic event in my life would appear much different to me now as an adult. It could quite possibly appear much less painful, and thus free the trauma that had accompanied and haunted me for these many years. As she and I went through this exercise, I realized that the event we reviewed actually had some funny parts to it. And although I hadn't seen any of that humor as a child, looking now through a new, adult frame, I found that I did.

I began thinking that maybe I had found my answer: the way for me to spend more of my time smiling, laughing, and being happy was to go back and reframe more of my personal stories. The key was that I would need to reframe the stories with a focus on finding something in the events that could be construed as funny. This wasn't going to be easy since the trauma still exists. It did not mean I had to try to change the story, as that would be impossible to do, but rather my *perception* of it. For example, I would have a choice: I could remain traumatized by remembering the time when I was three years old and my father was about to strike my brother and, while screaming and crying, I just stood there and did nothing, – *or* I could reframe the memory into a funny picture where this little kid attacks and tries to bring down his 200-plus-pound father!

The more I practiced reframing my traumatic experiences with humor, the easier it became. I started to realize that maybe I really had lived a pretty crazy (funny) life, and that perhaps others would appreciate hearing about it. So, I began to repeat my stories to my friends, reframing the events wherever I could to present them with as much humor as possible, and my friends responded the way I did: they laughed! The more stories I told, the more they laughed, and the more fun I had sharing. I was releasing those "feel-good" endorphins in my friends and in myself.

People *like to laugh*, and people *like to make others laugh* too. And, the good news is we don't have to be professional comedians to participate in the process: we just have to learn to look at situations and realize that we *can* reframe them. We can't change them as they occurred, but we can change the way they look to us. *We can consciously choose to use a lighter, less traumatic frame than the one that was there previously.* We all know how to laugh; we also know what makes us laugh. I've learned that when I make myself laugh, others around me laugh, too. It's kind of like yawning. It's pretty hard not to yawn when the lady next to you is yawning, isn't it? *The same goes with laughter...it's contagious!*

This book is about my struggles with mental illness, its stigma, and words that have hurt me. It's about me, and many of the traumas in my life, and how they have saddled me at times with severe pain and deep depression. But it's also about how I've learned to "unstick" many of those traumas – primarily by using my sense of humor to reframe them, to change the way they've been pictured in my head, so that they are not as frightening and debilitating as they had once been.

I did not write this book as proof that what I have learned to do has "cured" me. Mental illnesses such as depression are *biological* diseases (some say brain disorders). The truth is that I may always be in recovery, never able to be fully cured. Although my depression has been triggered at various times by different events and the behaviors of others toward me, my illness has always been "there." *It is also extremely important for me to understand that my illness isn't my fault;* I can't help the fact that I have this biological problem any more than I can help contracting any other disease. Look at how many people have never smoked cigarettes, yet have suffered from lung cancer. Is it their fault? And how about those who have discovered they have inherited a specific gene that causes certain cancers? We *can't* say it's their doing!

Why is it then that we don't blame ourselves for contracting some diseases, but the *biological* disease of mental illness carries with it such a stigma that many people refuse to seek treatment? So many of us are afraid and embarrassed. What would our friends, relatives, and co-workers think if they knew we were living with depression, bipolar disorder, ADHD, or another mental illness? As a result of the stigma, a tremendous number of people are not seeking the help they need, and so they aren't getting better, and are thus unable to manage their illnesses. This is not just devastating to the consumers themselves; this hurts all of us as we waste billions of dollars in health care costs that are out of control.

It is my hope that this book will serve several purposes: (1) I want it to be fun for you to read. As Will Rogers says above, go right ahead and laugh at all the crazy things that have happened to me, since they didn't happen to you! (2) I want to share with you how I have been able to recall traumatic events in my life and then reframe them so that I can now enjoy at least parts of them. (3) I want you to use me as a frame of reference, as someone who has been there, done that, AND has had a successful, relatively happy life with great friends and family. People living with a mental illness *can* and *do* succeed in all facets of life, and I'm just one example. (4) I hope you will begin to seek and learn the facts about mental illness: it is a *biological* disease, and as such it is not my fault that I have it. I also want for you to come to trust that I can learn to manage my mental illness. By understanding that most mental illnesses are manageable, you will be helping to reduce the terribly unwarranted and embarrassing stigma associated with it.

Enjoy the book and the zany stories from the life of a person living with depression who has discovered that reframing those stories can effectively reduce their trauma and debilitating pain.

Did I tell you yet about the time they cut me open like a chicken? See Chapter Three!

John Shuchart
April 2015

Introduction

"Insanity runs in my family. It practically gallops."
—Cary Grant

If the Hindus' belief in reincarnation is accurate, I would surmise that I'm at the stage in my current life cycle where I've spent the past sixty-six years as a deer in someone's headlights. This includes frantically deciding which direction I should move in order to save my life, and knowing that if I don't hurry and get out the way, my next cycle will find me adorning a wall in some hunter's trophy room!

My life has been one "are you kidding me?" episode after another. A few of those episodes have been so crazy that I just had to share them with *someone*, and thus, you the reader are hereby so anointed. The bizarreness of my life began as early as my conception, when my mother tried to drown me out of her womb. It continues to the present, as I anticipate a sixteenth surgery next month, the result of being T-boned by a guy hauling concrete blocks more than a decade ago. That's a depressing thought. And that's what this book is about, sort of .... It's really about my *living* with depression and the stigma that is unfortunately and tragically attached to it. The book is also about the many words that have hurt me through the years, creating traumas that have been stuck in my brain ever since hearing them. Finally, it's about the the Dark Hole of Depression, something that we who live with the disease fully understand, but others don't because they've never experienced it. The Hole is so dark and deep that it is extremely difficult to escape, and it is a place of despair and utter hopelessness. Those of us who have dwelled in the Hole believe that things with us are bad, will get worse, and will never, ever get better. The Hole can often tease us, using its power to make us think it is our protector. It tries to make us feel safe, free from the pressures of the outside. In the Hole, we don't have to move, we can curl up in the fetal position and not have to cope with what is really hurting us. I've learned that it is easier to remain *outside* the Hole than it is to escape from the inside, and by using humor, I can often times break my fall into the Hole. When I feel one of my depressive episodes coming on, I have a choice: I can let go and slip and slide downward, or I can apply the brakes by doing something that halts the ruminating going on in my head ("Johnny, you're a loser; things are horrible; they'll never get better; you're a terrible, rotten person.").

Recent studies have shown that if you can stop the negative chain of thought that accompanies depression, you can actually redirect your thought patterns, and thereby stop a depressive episode before it starts.. Using my sense of humor has become how I disrupt what's spinning around in my head. I have learned to laugh at myself and at the crazy things that have happened to me that I admit certainly weren't funny at the time. In fact, many were horribly traumatic. I mean, having a lawnmower, with the blade rotating, fall on top of me was not funny: but what the surgeon asked me when I awoke sure was! It also wasn't funny when my parents separated, but looking back, it makes me smile when I think of the way my father tried to bribe his way back into the family, and how his gift to me almost knocked me unconscious!

And speaking of family, mine was probably no better or worse than yours; it's just the one I know. The cast of characters includes three brothers and a set of heterosexual parents. My mother was extremely loving and nurturing. She was also in psychotherapy almost her entire adult life for a myriad of mental illnesses. She could at times be verbally abusive, especially with me, and later in life when she discovered the drink most favored by many Russians, she stepped into the role of a very mean drunk. She was raised by the greatest *people* in the world (my grandparents), but unfortunately not by the greatest *parents*. From what I have been told by aunts and uncles who were there, my grandparents never learned how to tell my mother anything other than "yes." When she was just a young kid around five or six years old, she supposedly told her father she wanted a pony, and a few days later she had one. My mother learned quickly: later in life she saw her sister-in-law with a new fur coat and told my father she wanted one too. My father supposedly told her "no," and the story goes that Mom went to her father to complain and, you guessed it: Mom had a nice new fur coat. There are many more instances I've heard of that are similar to these, but you get the point: Mom never knew what it was like to be without whatever it was that she wanted…until late in her life when my father's financial status suddenly changed, and for the first time ever, she found herself being asked to live within her means (whatever that meant).

I understand that it is difficult to drop social classes, especially several at a time — and in just a matter of weeks rather than years. My mother really did go from riches to rags in a hurry, and she never had the proper amount of time and help to make the adjustment. She had almost 100 percent of her assets stripped from her as her husband went from business owner and wealthy entrepreneur to an unemployed, unskilled, and defeated man. She went from living with almost no budget, to well, no budget, but for different reasons: one because she thought she had unlimited resources, and two, because she had none. For most of the time though, she lived in Never-Never Land as Mom continued to spend money she didn't have. No one on the planet went to the grocery store more often than she did (think four to five times each week). And no one ever hoarded more paper towels, toilet paper, paper plates, or packages of Wrigley's gum than my mother. She bought what she thought she needed and then bought more and then some more. She never bought *one* of anything, ever. She didn't have one or two cigarette lighters; she had four or five at all times. She had pantries and shelves full of everything you could imagine . . . well, every-thing you could imagine a grocery store stocking. I can't ever remember asking her, "Mom, do you have..." without the answer being, "yes, of course, let me get that for you!" She even stocked our friends' favorites, including their brands of cigarettes!

Mom's compulsive behavior was, of course, just that: compulsive. This issue wasn't limited to material goods, either. She was compulsive in her drinking later in life, her incessant talking on the phone, and her endless berating of my father. She was constantly tearing him down for being a loner, lazy, unloving, and a totally aloof person. The few times he would physically approach her with a warm, gentle hug, she would invariably push him away. It's ironic that as cold as she accused Dad of being, it was really she who preferred to stay at home, away from any physical or social interactions with him or anyone else.

Mom was no dummy: she read a lot (newspapers) and watched the news. She formed opinions quickly, but was disturbingly somewhat racist, and arrogant at times. She would have taken the time to learn how to use FaceTime, search the Internet, and Google everything under the sun had the technology been available, but whatever she would have mastered would never have changed her: she was convinced that the most important thing in the world was money. Without it, neither she nor anyone could be happy.

Two events in our household, outside of the old man going broke, changed everything forever: my father being robbed and shot, and my brother Steve's death. My father's escapade, which you'll be reading about later, had a profound effect upon my mother. It gave her too much time to sit and feel sorry for herself, and it triggered her bout with vodka. The primary result of her drinking was how it impacted her treatment of me. Steve was married, and my younger brothers, Fred and Jay, were in elementary school, so that left me to act as her punching bag. And, boy, could she hit hard. The words she spewed at me hurt; in fact, they're the basis of much of what follows in the book. I can't count the number of times I was told how horrible a person I was, that I would never amount to anything, that it was such a waste that I couldn't be more like Steve (this was before he killed himself), and on and on. For the most part I made sure I physically stood erect and took it, but emotionally I often crumbled. I was especially sensitive to the outrageous things she said about my future wife, Stevie, someone who always bent over backwards to be polite and kind to her. My mother was jealous of Stevie, jealous of the time I spent with her, and in essence, angry about the loss of control over her son she thought she was experiencing. In simple terms, my mother couldn't, *wouldn't* let go.

This certainly didn't seem to be the case as far as her feelings toward my father were concerned: she *always* acted like she wanted to let *him* go! Their marriage wasn't rocky; it wasn't tumultuous…it was a relationship of total mutual destruction. They spent hours on end verbally abusing each other: "Al, you are the worst! You can't talk to me or anyone else. You have NO feelings. What is wrong with you?!" And, of course, the rebuttal from Dad: "Jeanne, shut up! Get off that darn phone! You just yap and yap." I spent my entire youth listening to these and many more character assassinations as they tore each other down night after night.

If my father had been a "normal" man, he'd have either thrown the phone at Mom and killed her, or moved out and left. But, Dad was anything but "normal." Raised in a home without much warmth, he married my mother and admitted to me that he never thought about having a family. He never wanted kids (that was fun to hear him say). He once informed me that he had told my mother that, but that she had laughed it off and married him anyway. He was a father who picked his spots: he ate dinner with us, then usually proceeded to his place on the couch and stayed there until he either fell asleep or somehow managed to carry himself into his bedroom.

The only activity I can remember that ever got him off the couch consistently was when I was playing a sport, usually baseball. Unfortunately for me, his desire to control the game and his son meant that every year I played ball, he had to be my manager. Of course, I was never good enough, even though I was always the star of the team. If I was pitching, he would yell at me at the top of his lungs whenever my pitches missed the plate. He didn't care how much he embarrassed me, screaming at me like I was an idiot. Whenever I was batting, I didn't walk enough or hit enough homers; whenever I was catching, I didn't ever "call" a good game; and whenever the pitcher was getting clobbered, it was always because I wasn't holding the target in the right places.

You'll read more about Dad and his military ways, his inflexibility, and his temper in the pages that follow, but I think this quick story describes these traits pretty well. He was sent off to a military academy as a youth and learned that there were only three acceptable answers in life: "Yes, Sir!" "No, Sir!" and "No excuse, Sir!" If you're wondering exactly what that meant, one night my older brother, Steve, came home fifteen minutes after curfew. His hands, face, and clothes were filthy, and he said he was late because he had a flat tire, which he had obviously changed himself...a very un-Shuchart thing to do, by the way. While most parents would have quickly understood, empathy never crossed my father's mind. I swear that to this day, these were his exact words: "There is *no* excuse for *ever* being late. You should have left wherever you were with enough time to spare to make allowance for the *possibility* of a flat tire." Steve made the mistake of speaking, and my father smashed him in the jaw hard enough to help him lose some weight over the next couple of days, as he was restricted to sucking soup through a straw. *This* is the father I lived with.

As far as brother Steve was concerned, he was my idol. As younger brothers often do, I found myself chasing him wherever he ran, hoping he would let me play with him and his friends. Of course, that wasn't to be: Steve always thought of me as the "kid" and treated me as such. Although we came from the same parental units, we were as different as oil and water: me the extrovert, Steve the recluse. He spent more time as a teenager in his room eating popcorn, drinking Vess red soda, and reading science fiction books than doing much of anything else. He was always a one-friend and one-girlfriend at a time kind of person. He was extremely smart (think photographic memory if there is indeed such a thing), very handsome (think Nordic, blond hair, blue eyes), and could crush a golf ball (think 3 handicap). But, he was also lazy; things came too easily to him, and his outward, confident appearance ended up fooling us all, as he took his own life at age twenty-seven.

My mother gave birth to Steve about eighteen months after she was married, and then I arrived nineteen months later (much unwanted, as you'll soon discover in Chapter One). And, just when everyone assumed my parents had forsaken sex forever, eleven long and tumultuous years later, little bro Fred showed up, followed a couple of years later by yet another brother, Jay. By the time my younger brothers arrived, my parents had aged, and with aging comes change: they had either mellowed or had just plain worn out. They treated this second generation of little Shucharts with a much gentler hand. I'm not saying things were perfect for my younger brothers, but from what I could tell when I looked into their storage unit and discovered more baseball gloves and balls and cleats and whatnot than I could've possibly imagined my father ever buying me, I knew something had changed in the household where I grew up. I wasn't around the family much during those years, as I had escaped to college, and with the large disparity in our ages, I never really developed much of a relationship with either of the "kids." They're grown now, each successful attorneys with families of their own. We've gone our separate ways, me with my glove and each of them with their own caches.

I'm excited to share my life's adventures with you, and even though they will most certainly draw some significant laughs, there's a serious message or two that I hope to successfully convey. First, my mental illness of depression is not my fault, that I didn't do anything to get it, and there is *nothing* I could have done to prevent it. (Mental illness has been proven to be a brain disorder.) Second, even though I have done nothing wrong, my illness carries with it a horrible, painful stigma. Each of us who lives with a mental illness is subject to ridicule, blame, and often times worse. Many of us, especially young people, feel so embarrassed and stigmatized that we refuse to seek the help we need, fearing that doing so will expose our illnesses to friends and relatives who will then shun us. This doesn't need to be the case. *People with mental illnesses can and do succeed; this book is proof of that as it relates to me. Hey, I've written a book! I've had a successful business career. I've got a great family and some pretty wonderful friends. I have served on numerous nonprofit boards and have developed important projects for youth at risk, all while struggling with serious bouts of depression. Mental illness does not have to be an impediment to one's success any more than any other disease.* I believe that. I'm hopeful that you will, too.

Enjoy the book, laugh along with me, and join in the fight to end the stigma. Become a member of your local chapter of the National Alliance on Mental Illness (NAMI). Contact the Greater Kansas City Coalition on Mental Illness (www.itsOK.us) about starting your own local coalition. And don't forget your sense of humor. Using it will help you help yourself, and others, from ever experiencing the Dark Hole of Depression.

A man's got to take a lot of punishment to write a really funny book."
—Ernest Hemingway

Chapter 1

"I have to get rid of this kid, *NOW!*"

"I could tell my parents hated me.
My bath toys were a toaster and a radio."
—Rodney Dangerfield

My therapist tells me that the very first words I ever heard from my mother were the triggers for my lifelong struggle with depression. I was only a couple of minutes into my existence when Mom started screaming hysterically. My conception had just occurred. This was a miracle in itself since my parents had sex about as often as the Kansas City Royals make the baseball playoffs. My mother must have had a premonition, because she jumped out of bed and ran toward the bathroom shrieking, "Quick, Al, get your ass up and help me run a bath! I HAVE GOT TO GET RID OF THIS KID, *NOW!*"

(At least I think that's what she screamed.[1] I hadn't developed anything resembling a sense of hearing yet, so I may have misunderstood some of what was said at the time. However, since we're taking a lot of license in this first chapter, I ask for your indulgence and use of your imagination as the story unfolds.)

Talk about words that hurt! What a way to start my life. I wasn't even an inch long and there my mother was trying everything she could to wash me away! What did she think I was? Chopped liver? Swiss cheese? Burnt toast?

In spite of her best efforts, I survived. But knowing that your mother doesn't want you sticks in your brain *forever*. I mean, mom is probably the most important person in your life (you think your *father* would carry you around for nine months?). We spend forever trying to please her, trying to gain her unconditional support and love. So, to learn my mother didn't want me, and actually tried to do me in, was and is, incredibly traumatic.

As a result of Mom's furious attempt to eliminate me, I spent a lot of my time in her womb wondering just what was so terrible about keeping me around for the next 85 years or so. My parents had wanted to wipe me out before they ever had a clue who I was, or what I'd become. Whatever happened to that Spanish saying, *qué será, será*? Didn't they at least want to know what I would look like before they zapped me? What if I was going to become a doctor or lawyer (*every* Jewish mother's dream for her son)? Or maybe I might discover a cure for cancer or mental illness. Perhaps I'd become the first Jewish professional football player that anyone actually

---

[1] I've read that researchers have discovered that while we're floating around in the womb, we can actually hear the things that are going on outside. Supposedly we are able to feel the vibrations created by the noise and are able to somehow distinguish between Mom telling us how much she loves us and Dad begging for *you know what*. I recreated my conception and first six and a half months in the womb shortly after the first time my mother told me the story about her trying to get rid of me immediately after conception. I'm sharing the story exactly as I have always thought it probably went down had I really been able to know what was happening around me.

remembers! And as for Dad, his dream was to have a great athlete in the family, someone who could excel in several sports but especially in baseball. What was it that made my parents so determined not to have another kid—to wipe me out before I had the chance to play Madden NFL 15 on Xbox?

One of their reasons, I figured out later, was that they already had a child—my brother Steve, who was about a year old at the time. And the last thing they wanted was a Steve II. Named after absolutely nobody, Steve's big mistake, as far as I could make out, was that he looked nothing like Dad. The old man thought Steve's skin was far too fair to adequately represent the Shuchart side of the family, and given that Steve's hair was as blond as the best Norwegian could ever hope for, it was obvious that he looked like one of "them," the Wises, my mother's side of the family. Or, perhaps our fair-haired mailman. Either way, Dad didn't want much to do with little Steve and certainly wasn't anxious to have another Norwegian running around our apartment.

So after my mother sprang out of bed, she dashed into the bathroom, long-jumped into the bathtub, and began the process of trying to make brother Steve an only child. She screamed for Dad to help her turn on the water, but he was already sound asleep. (It's what guys do after sex...sleep.) I was surprised our neighbors in the building didn't come running to help her. Her shrills must have awakened more than a few of them; it sure got my attention, all those ghastly vibrations it caused in her uterus.

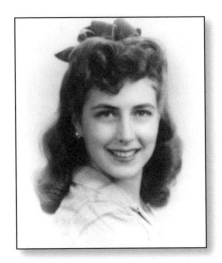

What a fox Mom was! Why aren't I gorgeous, too?

It turns out that whatever Mom tried in the name of "getting rid of this kid NOW" didn't work. It also didn't leave me feeling all that thrilled about my prospects. So, taking no chances, I decided my best shot at survival was to flee. I figured if I got out of wherever I was, it would be harder for my parents to finish me off. My plan was simple: with about six weeks still to go, I'd start kicking and punching as hard as I could and hope for the best.

When the time came, I was ready. I began my journey by flipping myself upside down (I had heard somebody, I think it was Aunt Hermia, talking one time about a "breech birth" and, after hearing her describe it, I was all in for a head-first exit). I couldn't figure out how I was going to escape, though; my head seemed gargantuan compared to the teeny, tiny escape hatch near my crown. After giving it some thought, I figured that if my brother Steve had made it so could I. Closing my eyes and holding my breath, I began kicking and clawing as hard and fast as I could. Nothing. Nada. I got nowhere. I heard lots of garbled voices, some louder than others, but none as loud as Mom's. She wasn't talking; she was shrieking again. It couldn't be anything I was doing, could it? Maybe she was on to my plan, my Great Escape. Yep, that's definitely what was happening. She realized I wanted out, and she was in no way happy about the thought of me making it into the world.

This scenario—me kicking, Mom screaming—went on from early in the evening into the wee hours of the next day. By that time I was pooped. I remember thinking that Steve must have been the *strongest* kid ever to be able to escape. As for me, in between episodes of kicking here, clawing there, I managed to get some shut-eye. When morning came I must have rolled over or pushed on something, because at about nine o'clock I was awakened by yet another horrific scream from my Mom: "If you don't get this kid out NOW, I'm going to die! Do SOMETHING and do it FAST!"

This was my wake up call. With more determination than ever, I started pushing with my legs and grabbing anything I could find with my hands. I turned my head just enough to catch a faint light shining above me. It was coming from the escape hatch, but the hatch itself was still too small for me to fit through. Just as I started to wonder again how Steve ever made it out, the light suddenly increased to the point that my home for the past several months lit up like a Christmas tree! I looked up and, squinting my tiny eyes, was able to see that the escape hatch had widened, and I found myself looking at a bunch of really huge people, and a room so bright I thought it was that light everyone claims to see after they die. *Was I dead? Had I entered the World to Come?*

No such luck. I was still about to enter into *this* world. Within seconds of my arrival, just after my entire body had been yanked into *this* world, some really big person grabbed me and put me on top of someone else. This, I was soon to discover, was dear old Mom. No one told me she was Mom, but it quickly became pretty obvious. Upon seeing me lying there on her belly, she started screaming—no, shrieking— again, and I immediately recognized *that* sound for myself!

I'll never forget my first glance at her face. Her eyes were swollen, her cheeks bright red, and her hair all tangled in sweat-soaked dreadlocks or something. I didn't need Dr. Phil to tell me I was looking at the face of an extremely disappointed person. Had she wanted a girl, maybe? Nah, that couldn't be it. After all, this was the woman who had tried everything she could to get rid of me before there was any chance of knowing my sex.

As disappointed as Mom was that I came out, she was, on top of that, frustrated to no end that I had decided to make my appearance six weeks early. Back in the Stone Age when I was born, preemies like me had to remain in the hospital for weeks before they were allowed to go home. Turns out that I was so fragile (weighing in at three and one-half pounds) that it bought me a whole month's stay. I lived in an incubator in the nursery where babies by the score were coming and going each day, but not *moi*. I just lay there, usually on my stomach, looking at my hands all day, wondering what they were and what I was supposed to be doing with them.

From where my incubator was I couldn't quite see the old analog clock on the wall in the nursery, so I didn't know how many days or weeks I had been banished to this life of eating, sleeping, pooping, repeat, but one day Mom showed up. By sheer luck, I had been rolled over on my back by some careless nurse (who would have gotten a medal these days for saving me from SIDS), so I was able to see Mom standing against the glass that separated me from the rest of the world. She was crying. I figured she was so happy to see me—and the progress I was making—that she just couldn't hold back her tears. Instead, she was bawling as she began to face the reality that little Johnny would soon be released to be an occupant in her apartment, as well as her life.

The big day came about five weeks after the Great Escape. The nurses delivered the devastating news to my parents: "There is nothing further we can do for your boy...it's time for you to take him home." They placed me in my mother's arms, stuck a pacifier in my mouth to shut me up, and wheeled us both down the hall toward the exit doors. I was a little baffled as to why they had my mother sit in a wheelchair; was there something wrong with her legs? I knew I couldn't walk, but what was *her* problem? Could it be that I was now part of a mentally *and* physically challenged family?

When we arrived at the hospital's exit, I finally met my father. He was leaning against our car, holding onto a cigarette, his eyes focused on the ground in front of him. The nurse pushing our wheelchair took me from Mom and turned to hand me to the old man, who, after taking a deep drag on his unfiltered Chesterfield, turned toward my mother and barked, "Take YOUR kid, Jeanne. I want nothing to do with him." Ouch! Words that hurt! Didn't he read the books?

Didn't he know that even though I couldn't read or write, I could still feel the bad vibrations emanating from this Sephardic-looking man?

And so, the fighting about me between my parents had begun. My father spent the rest of his life blaming my mother for not being able to drown me, and my mother blamed my father for wanting to have sex in the first place.

For the drive home, somebody was going to have to hold me (car seats hadn't been invented yet), but my two prospects were fighting, and it was obvious neither one wanted to be stuck with me. Dad walked over to the driver's side, got in, and slammed his door so hard the windows almost broke. After Mom got into the car, the nurse put me into her arms and closed her door, but before Mom could get a firm grip on me, the old man floored it, and we took off like a rocket. Somehow Mom managed to keep me from flying through the rear window. I was so grateful that I left her a Surprise. Yep, you got it—I did number one and number two. The force of our takeoff somehow caused my diaper to rip from one of the pins (disposable diapers hadn't been invented yet), leaving my bottom quite naked. Poor Mom was covered with my Surprise. She looked at my father and was speechless. He looked back at her and let her have it. "That's it! That kid is going to be a pain in the ass forever. Good going, Jeanne. I hope you're happy. Another kid—just want we didn't need."

And that's how my life started—as just another "kid we didn't need."

How I've reframed my beginning...

What you've just read is, in fact, how I've reframed my beginning. By making my entire experience from conception to coming home from the hospital somewhat ludicrous and funny (we know that most of what transpires in the story is my imaginative take on it), I've reframed the events. The truth is my mother really *did* try to wash me away; she took great pride in reminding me of this fact often through the years. I actually did show up some six weeks early as a preemie and had to remain in the hospital for almost five weeks before I weighed enough to be released. My father really did blame my mother for, well, almost everything that ever went wrong in their lives. And me? Well, I was often touted as their single biggest mistake.

Words hurt, especially words from your parents. I spent the better part of my life traumatized by knowing I was a "mistake." I guess I've had the opposite feelings of someone who is adopted. An adopted kid's biological parents may not want him, but his "real" parents do, and that goes a long way toward covering any wounds. In my case, I didn't have anywhere else to go for comfort, so I carried this trauma of rejection for a long time.

My sense of humor in reframing this story has helped me "unstick" what I've gone through. I laughed a lot while writing this chapter. And when I can connect laughter to the story, the truth doesn't seem to hurt as much. It's hard to laugh and cry at the same time.

I hope you read this chapter with a grin, and maybe even laughed some. If you did, then arm yourself with this chapter. File it away somewhere in your brain so you can bring it to mind whenever you need a reason to smile. Better yet, create your own story of your birth. Put yourself in the womb; give yourself a mouth, ears, and whatnot and try to hear what others were saying while you wiled away the nine months. I bet your story is pretty funny!

Chapter 2

"Where are the goldfish?"

"The most remarkable thing about my mother is that for thirty years she served the family nothing but leftovers. The original meal has never been found."
—Calvin Trillin

Miraculously, I survived the ride from the hospital. The home to which I was taken was an old apartment, one of many in a huge building situated right in the middle of a Jewish Ghetto—also known as the Moorlands in Clayton, Missouri. My room? Well, I didn't really have one, at least not until later when I became my brother's roommate; he never forgave me for that...nor for being born.

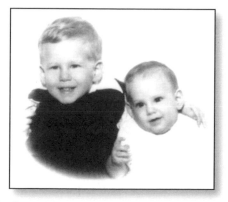

The "Nordic" Steve and me, at age 10 months

I had a table with a pad on it that sat in the hallway just outside Steve's door. I guess the folks were hoping their two-year-old would take care of me—jump up when I cried, change my diaper, feed me a bottle, and tell me when to shut up and go to sleep.

Nothing special happened over the next couple of years, at least nothing that I can remember. Trouble did arise when I was about two years old. My parents separated. It wasn't that surprising, since they argued and screamed at each other a lot. They each had a special way of setting the other off. The one thing that drove my father crazy was that my mother never shut up. She talked on our one black, extremely heavy, rotary-dial Southwestern Bell telephone for hours on end. She was unbelievable. She could cook, set the table, lay out our clothes, brush our teeth—all while talking on the phone. This amazing talent, however, went very much unappreciated by Dad. "Jeanne, get off the phone!" he'd scream at the top of his lungs. "You've been on it for hours!" My mother would reply, just as loudly, "Why, you expecting a call? Nobody calls for you, Al. Nobody *likes* you!"

For my part, I remember being pretty impressed that Mom could multitask, especially since Dad could only do one thing at a time—either yell at us, watch our eight-inch black-and-white television from about five inches away, read the paper, or fart and look around for who did it. Whenever I would teeter up to him and ask, "What's that smell?" he would ask me if I had pooped in my diaper. I would come to find out that nothing was ever that man's fault.

When the time came for the folks to tell us about the big separation, my father was AWOL. Mom had Steve and me sit back on our incredibly ugly couch with the thick, sticky and at the same time slippery, vinyl cover. My family and everyone we knew encased each piece of their furniture in this obnoxious plastic, making sitting extremely uncomfortable but preserving the furniture for future generations. Mom got down on one knee in front of us and very seriously and somewhat sternly said she had something very important to tell us.

"Your dad is moving out of the house. He's moving to a place called Tulsa."

Tulsa? What—and where—was that? Did all dads go there at one time or another? Well, if that was where he was headed, I hoped he was walking there—we only had one car and we needed it! I looked at Steve, and he was smiling. He knew the old man didn't like him; Steve was too Norwegian-looking. He figured with my father out of the house, life would be better.

My reaction was quite different. I was traumatized. I remember crying and asking why Dad was leaving, not letting on that my real issue was with Mom—as in, why wasn't *she* leaving too? She told me Daddy still loved me (who was she kidding?) and that he would be back every now and then to visit, blah, blah, blah. Unlike Steve, I wondered what part I might be playing in Dad's departure. I mean, Mom and Dad fought about the telephone, but they also fought about us kids. Funny thing was, they fought mostly about Steve, but I was the one who was most bothered by their arguments.

Whatever Dad's reasons were for leaving, I remember being really sad and scared, and my mother sensed it. I asked her about our car. "Well, Daddy is moving to Tulsa like I just told you and he needs our car," she began. "It's really far away, and I'm afraid he can't live there without it. So we won't have a car, but we'll be okay. Grandpa will drive us wherever we need to go, I promise."

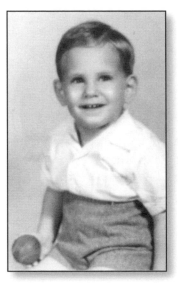

Here's me at two years old, around the time Dad split for Tulsa

Grandpa Wise's driving record was such that the Cadillac dealership had a new car sitting on their lot with his name on it at all times. You see, Grandpa was a fairly heavy man and had trouble turning his neck. He could sometimes look right or left, but glancing behind while backing up was a crapshoot. Maybe in another era it wouldn't have been such a big deal, but we're talking about the 1950s when the typical Caddy had huge fins on the back. Grandpa would invariably smash his taillights two or three times a month. In fact, Grandpa had no trouble smashing other parts of his car too. He almost killed himself a couple of times while running red lights at intersections. He would jump out of his smashed car and start screaming at the guy he creamed, "You idiot! What are you doing? I had a yellow light, and you're smashing into me!?" It was *red*, trust me. The cops would give Grandpa a ticket, another to add to his glove box that was full of them, and then he would call the Cadillac dealership to come exchange his car for a new one.

Somehow we survived without the old man *and* the car. We mooched rides from Grandpa when we needed to, but we kept that to an absolute minimum to avoid the risk of long hospital stays. The new arrangement didn't last for long, though. Six months later, we found out Daddy was returning home.

By that time, I was potty trained, so my father could no longer blame his farts on me. I was also talking up a storm, though not up to Mom's standards, and running everywhere I needed to go. I had adjusted to life without Dad quite well. It hadn't been rocket science. I didn't really miss him. After all, he had never gotten up to take me to bed or change my diaper, *ever*, so other than seeing him at dinner and watching him watch our eight-inch television, there wasn't much for me to miss. But just as I'd had no say in his leaving, nobody asked me about letting him come back, either.

For some reason the old man wanted to make his return a big deal. As we were eating another of those horrible Swanson's TV dinners, which was about as gourmet as Mom got, the old man walked out of their bedroom. He looked the same, but he sure didn't act like the angry, out-of-control, farting father that left us six months ago. He was smiling, and he even kissed me! It was really bizarre. I mean, it had to have been if I still remember it. And then came the coup de grâce…Dad said he had a "surprise" for us if we ate our dinners. That reminded me of the last surprise he had given us—taking the car and leaving us in the perilous hands of Grandpa Wise. Steve rolled his eyes, moved what was left of his Swiss steak to cover up the hard-as-gravel green peas, and began to eat the hearty apple pie dessert that had been surgically placed by the Swanson people into the top left-hand square of the TV dinner tray.

Being a toddler, I didn't really care about the past—I wanted the surprise! I quickly finished the yucky parts of my dinner, even deciding to forgo the pie. I got down from my booster chair and looked up at my dad, wondering where he was hiding whatever he was planning on presenting us with. He turned to Steve, who was still playing with his cool Swanson aluminum tray, and told him to get down from the table, wash his hands, and join us as soon as possible. Again, Steve rolled his eyes. He was smart enough to know whatever awaited us was a scam of sorts and reluctantly headed toward the bathroom to wash up. I went into our living room, actually holding the old man's hand, and waited for Steve. Even Mom hung up the phone for once and ditched her apron to join us. I've always wondered why this woman needed an apron to heat up TV dinners…

When we were all uncomfortably seated on our vinyl-encased living room couch, Dad announced that he had some really great gifts for us, and we would need to sit quietly while he slipped into the bedroom to retrieve them. I remember sitting on the edge of the couch, being stuck to the vinyl as if glued there, eagerly waiting to grab whatever was coming my way. Steve, on the other hand, was slouched way back in the couch, his arms folded with an "Okay, impress me" look on his face. After a few seconds the old man reappeared, holding in each hand what looked like fishbowls.

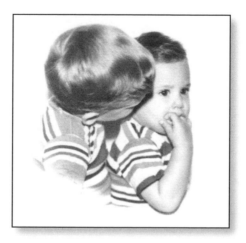

Steve can't believe I am sucking my middle two fingers!

"Wow, cool," exclaimed Steve, struggling to slide off the couch and showing some emotion for the first time that night. "Where are the goldfish?"

"Eh, goldfish? There aren't any goldfish, son. These are spacesuits—space helmets."

"What's a space helmet?" asked Steve. "I don't think I want a space helmet. Let's just do the goldfish."

Dad was already getting frustrated, which was nothing new, and definitely not something we had all missed for the past six months. "Steve, I told you. This is a space helmet. You put it over your head when you're on Mars. It helps you breathe."

Mars? What was the old man talking about? How would any of us know what Mars was? I was two and Steve was almost four. Mom popped TV dinners into the oven, talked all day on the phone, and wouldn't know what a Mars was if it hit her in the face.

"When are we going to this Mars?" Steve asked. "And I thought you said something about a spacesuit. Where's that part of the surprise?"

"Just a minute and I'll get it. Now, when you're on Mars you will need to wear the suit as well as the helmet. You see, the atmosphere on Mars isn't the same as it is on Earth, so you'll need these special outfits in order to help you breathe."

That did it. I was about to ask a question, but Steve interrupted. "Okay, I think I just want the goldfish. I don't really want to go to Mars."

Naturally, I seconded Steve's motion. I had no clue about this Mars thing and didn't know much more about goldfish, but I figured that if Steve was pushing for them, they must be better than going to someplace where we couldn't breathe without a fishbowl on our heads.

The old man didn't know what to say. He went and got the spacesuits, and as soon as Mom saw them, she cracked up. She laughed so hard she started burping, and then wheezing, and finally crying. "Al, you have got to be kidding me! *Those* are spacesuits? Where did you get them? At Goodwill? And those helmets—Steve's right. Where are the goldfish? They're definitely fishbowls! What planet were you on when you bought them?"

While Mom laughed and Steve waited for the goldfish that would never come, I picked up my fishbowl, er, helmet, and put it over my head. It was so big and heavy that it plopped down and smacked the top of my head so hard I began to tear up. Even worse, after a few seconds I realized there were no holes in the helmet; there was no way for air to get into or out of it. When my breathing caused it to fog up, I got scared and started screaming. My mom reached down and pulled the bowl off my head, drew me toward her, and tried to comfort me. I could tell she was really angry.

"Great going, Al. Are you crazy? Why would you think they would want spacesuits, anyway? They have no clue what they are. How would they play with them?

The old man was speechless, but not without emotion. I could see him getting angry. His eyes became really small and focused; he pursed his lips, and his arms and hands tightened. He picked up the suits and the helmets and, without saying a word, walked out the front door, not even bothering to close it behind him.

Was he going back to Tulsa? Or maybe to Mars?

Reframing Breathing on Mars

Obviously, it's no picnic when parents separate. It affects everyone involved—the parents, the kids, the in-laws, the out-laws, maybe even the dogs and the cats (goldfish, too?). Even though I was so young when the the first of several separations happened, I know it hurt and confused me. I'm sure I was probably somewhat relieved and excited when my dad finally returned home, but probably my happiness was more about getting a surprise gift than having him return to the fold.

Whenever I retell this story, the biggest laughs come when people picture these two little kids (Steve and me) looking at those "helmets" with what had to be the most confused and disappointed faces. It's no fun to get a gift that you can't understand, can't really play with, and that might even hurt you (think heavy fishbowl crashing onto your head!). And to think my dad really thought we'd be excited about how important these spacesuits were going to be when we visited Mars. As my mother asked, what planet was he on?

I've learned to laugh at my father's feeble attempt to win the family back (because it's funny), but I've also gained some appreciation for his desire to try. As I grew older, I rarely if ever saw him show any emotion or affection toward me. He hugged and kissed my mother occasionally, but I don't have many recollections of him embracing me. So, his gesture of the spacesuits was probably something that was quite difficult for him. I know I only received two more presents from him from that day on (ones which came from him and not from both of my parents). One was a stamp catalogue (I started collecting stamps around fifth grade) and the other was a box of a dozen baseballs when I was in middle school. I had won some baby chickens at a carnival and he threw them away without telling anyone. My mother made him feel so guilty he had to do something to get out of her chicken house, er, doghouse!

Speaking of chickens, if you think my father's brain was on another planet at this point, it must have been really out to lunch when I had my appendix removed. That's next!

Chapter 3

"They're going to cut you open like a chicken."

*"I know that you believe you understand what you think
I said, but I'm not sure you realize that what you heard
is not what I meant."*
—Robert McCloskey

I was about five years old when I came down with what felt like a terrible stomachache. It was mostly on my right side. I told Mom about it and of course she was on the phone at the time, so she didn't pay much attention to what I was trying to tell her. I don't know with whom she was talking or how important the call was, I just knew I had an ache and it needed her attention.

In Mom's defense, she probably thought my pain was imaginary. You see, I was a bona fide hypochondriac. She knew, Dad knew, even Steve knew. Whenever something came up I didn't want to do, I got a stomachache. I used that particular physical impairment for quite a while, and when that stopped working for me, I switched to another one (earaches were pretty successful for me). Sometimes I faked a symptom so well that even I started believing I was suffering.

This particular time, though, was different. The pain in my side was real.

So Mom understandably blew me off and returned to her phone call. I remember stepping back to watch her, trying to think of a way to get her attention. She was sitting far away from where our old, black, rotary dial telephone was plugged into the wall. The cord was stretched to its limit, hanging about two feet off the ground. As Mom continued to babble away, I walked up to the cord and tried to step over it, thinking if I got closer to her she'd stop talking. I raised my leg about a foot into the air and suddenly felt like I had been stabbed in the side with a knife. I let out a short but very loud shriek, which really startled her.

"Excuse me, Lois, Johnny is screaming about something. Let me call you back."

"What is wrong with you?" She demanded as she slammed the phone down. "Can't you see I was on a phone call? Don't do that again! Now go play with something and leave me alone!"

"But, Mom, this time I'm not faking. There's some really big pain in my side. It really hurts!"

She looked at me as if she almost believed me. She asked me to raise my leg again to see if the pain would resurface, and sure enough it did. She turned back to the phone and took it off the receiver, but after a few seconds put it back. She was obviously thinking about what she should do. Meanwhile, I had decided to try lying down, so I walked ever so gingerly to our couch (the one with the yucky plastic cover on it) and tried to pull myself onto it. No luck. I kept first slipping and then sticking. Finally, I just lay down on the floor assuming the fetal position.

When Mom saw me lying there, she told me she was calling the doctor. Now normally, whenever she threatened to make that call, I would either retract my illness or, at a minimum, tell her that it wasn't "that bad"—that I was suddenly feeling better. But this time I didn't say a word, and she made the call.

My pediatrician was Max Deutch, a fifty-something-year-old balding guy who always—and I mean *always*—wore a coat *and* a tie. Either he didn't know he was supposed to wear a white smock or he simply refused to go along with convention, but he certainly never looked the part of a pediatrician. He had a really deep voice, and although he looked and sounded like a pretty intimidating guy, I never felt afraid of him. I think he always wanted to be the good cop, too, because he never gave me a shot; he always left that up to one of his nurses.

When Mom told Dr. Deutch about my side, he evidently didn't like what he heard, because as soon as they hung up, she told me he would be coming over to take a look at me. (If you're under the age of fifty-five you won't believe it when I tell you this, but doctors actually used to make house calls). Mom was no longer angry with me for interrupting her phone call, and in fact she was now doing whatever she could to console me. She helped me up onto the couch and sat next to me, gently rubbing my back. Every couple of minutes she'd ask me how I felt, and I really didn't know how to answer. I mean this was *real* pain.

Dr. Deutch showed up wearing, of course, his usual uniform. He sat down next to me and asked me where the pain was, and after touching my right side immediately stood up and walked my mother into the kitchen. When they reappeared, Dr. Deutch said he'd see me later and left. I asked my mother why I was hurting so much and she said Dr. Deutch wanted me to go to the hospital.

About an hour later my father showed up and took a suitcase out of the hall closet. Mom started bringing some of my clothes out of my room, mostly things like pajamas. Then it hit me that I might be *really* sick. A short time later, Steve and Grandpa Wise walked in (I guess it was late afternoon by that time, and Grandpa had picked up Steve at school). I knew if Grandpa was over without Grandma, something big had to be up. I learned later that she was already at the hospital waiting for us to arrive.

The next thing I remember was lying in a bed in my hospital room. A nurse was there and she was talking with my parents. After a few minutes, some big, strong guy came in and told me he was going to take me for a ride. Up until now I hadn't been scared, but for some reason this guy frightened me. My father must have realized I was becoming anxious, because as I was being wheeled out, he made sure I would know that he was going to walk alongside me. *Big* mistake!

Now at that time there was a show on television called *Medic*. I never really watched it (in those prehistoric days kids didn't watch much TV except for *Howdy Doody*), but occasionally I would glance at it whenever it was playing on the TV in our living room. I didn't understand much about what was going on in the show, but I *did* know that many times they would be pushing someone in a hospital bed just like mine down a long hallway. Eventually, they would stop, and there in front of them were these great big doors that would magically seem to open themselves. The bed would go through the doors and totally disappear . . . and *you never, ever saw anybody come back out again!*

Now I was in a hospital bed being pushed down a hall. The big guy was at my head pushing me along, while my father kept pace walking next to us so he could talk to me. I don't remember anything he said except for when we stopped in front of *those great big doors.* Leaning over my bed's railing, almost touching his nose to mine, he told me very matter-of-factly . . .

"They're going to cut you open like a chicken."

Huh? What? *Cut me open like a chicken?* Were they going to eat me, too? Needless to say, I went berserk. I started screaming and kicking my legs so hard that both the sheet and the blanket went flying into the air. The big guy grabbed me and pinned me down while two or three nurses came running out to help strap me down. Finally, they subdued me and began pushing me through the doors. Remembering what I had seen on *Medic*—that nobody ever came back once those doors closed—I went from being scared to *terrified.* At age five, I understood very little about surgery, and here I was about to be operated on—"cut open like a chicken." I went from kicking and screaming to scheming. I looked all around to see how I could get out when and if they unstrapped me. Maybe I could I play dead and then jump up and run away?

The next thing I knew, someone put a big rubber mask on my face. That did it! I resumed my kicking and screaming, but I was still pinned down. A few seconds later, they started sprinkling something into my mask. It smelled terrible. Little did I know that it was the knockout punch.

The next thing I remember was waking up back in my hospital room. My parents were there, and as I started to move they both came to my bedside and asked how I was doing. I answered: "Did they really cut me open like a chicken?"

My father just nodded. ARGH!

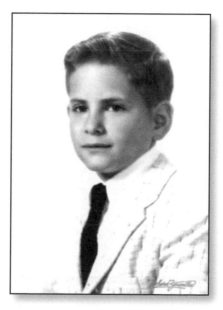

Age 5, shortly after I was "cut open like a chicken."

Reframing the Clucking

This was probably *the* most traumatic experience of my young life. My parents hadn't prepared me very well. They didn't tell me much about why I was in the hospital, and they didn't tell me where that big, frightening guy was taking me when he rolled my bed out of the room. My only knowledge of what was happening was supplied by my father. And telling me I was about to be cut open like a chicken was certainly not what anyone— regardless of age—would have wanted to hear.

As I look back on this episode in my life, after some sixty-one years have elapsed, I have to shake my head in disbelief at what my father said to me. It was so out of place, so crazy and irresponsible that I just have to smile. . .while also taking a deep breath. Try it for yourself right now. Repeat what he said: "They're going to cut you open like a chicken." I bet you said it and then shook *your* head too, just like I do. Your next words to yourself are probably something like, "hard to believe, amazing, *insane!*"

Words hurt, even when they're said in good faith. My father was an awkward man, socially inept, and had a difficult time communicating his feelings. I'm sure he was very uncomfortable walking beside my gurney, and figured he had to say *something*. In his mind, what he ended up blurting out was meant to be funny. Unfortunately, it wasn't, and it added to what was already a most traumatic event for me.

I'll never forget what the old man said, and how it demonstrated how socially awkward he was . . . but, I have learned to reframe all of this, to change how the picture looks to me. Instead of cringing whenever I pass a Popeyes restaurant, I usually start laughing as I imagine my father working there, cutting open a bunch of chicken breasts!

Chapter 4

"I think you have a right brain, left brain problem."

"We are all born ignorant, but one must work hard to remain stupid."
—Benjamin Franklin

My eleventh year of life was one of my most bizarre. First, as a Jewish youngster, I *should* have been preparing to become a Bar Mitzvah. Most of my Jewish friends began their Bar Mitzvah studies by attending Hebrew classes after school once or twice a week. The goal was to learn Hebrew and the prayers in the prayer book so they could lead the congregation in a service when they became an adult (age thirteen in the Jewish religion).

But they were studying; I wasn't. You see, at the time, I attended a private school. My mother said I flunked the school's entrance exam, but because Steve was already a brilliant student there, she was able to talk the school into accepting me. Anyway, classes got out each day at 4:45 p.m., but Hebrew schools usually started around 3:30 p.m., right after the public schools let out. My mother said she explained the problem to our rabbi and offered to pay for Steve and me to be privately tutored. "No way," he said. "All Bar Mitzvah candidates must attend Hebrew school together; I will not allow anyone to be privately tutored." I guess the synagogue was doing well and didn't need to host another couple of ceremonies.

At first, this didn't seem so bad. Most kids hated Hebrew school. Going to classes *after* regular school made for a really long day. Plus, studying Hebrew wasn't as much fun as going outside and playing Wiffle ball. But the reward was the actual Bar Mitzvah service, followed by a party and many, many presents. Over time, not being a Bar Mitzvah bothered me, not just because of the lost gifts but also because each of my own children eventually attended Hebrew school and participated in all the good things that happen when the ordeal ends. I'm proud to say that when I was almost fifty years old I decided to become a Bar Mitzvah. I knew the studying would be difficult at my advanced age, but since it was something my kids had done I felt I should honor them by following in their footsteps. This time there was no one to stop me from being tutored, and after a year or so of intense study, I became a Bar Mitzvah. It would have never happened without my Rabbi, Paul Silbersher, and my accountant, Jeff Marks, who spent almost every Tuesday afternoon with me for a full year, teaching me Hebrew and the prayers. To this day I'm not quite sure what motivated them to help me out so much (and for free), but I wouldn't have made it without them. When the big day came, I had a lot of fun leading the congregation, which included friends and family. Even my folks showed up! Afterwards, I finally got my big Bar Mitzvah party, but I'm *still* searching for the presents and money I would have gotten when I was thirteen. My take for my Bar Mitzvah was zilch!

Otherwise, I was a typical youngster on the cusp of becoming an acne-filled teenager. That meant my hormones were starting to play tricks on me, one day putting me in a good mood, the next day, not so much. I admit I was a handful, but I still don't think I deserve what was to happen next.

It started innocently enough at dinner one night. My mother asked me to pass her the salt, which I did. Then she said that she noticed I picked it up and passed it with my right hand. I replied that I was right-handed (she already knew that), so why would I use my other hand?

"I think you have a right brain, left brain problem," she said. "I've done some reading, and I think the reason you're struggling in school is because you are thinking out of the right side of your brain and writing right-handed. From what I've been reading, you should be writing with your *left* hand, because your brain waves and the hand you write with should *cross* each other. So if you were naturally left-handed like Dad, you would want to write right-handed instead. Come to think of it Al, you *do* write right-handed. See, Johnny, Dad is doing it the way it's supposed to be done."

The old man had this most quizzical look on his face, which told me that this was the first he had heard of Mom's newest theory on what was wrong with Johnny. "Jeanne, what on earth are you talking about? The kid is right-handed, period. Leave him alone. And for your information, I write right-handed because in school they hit me with a ruler any time I picked up a pencil with my left hand. They made everyone write with their right hand. This is crazy—drop it and just eat your dinner."

Mom didn't drop it, as usual. "Al, come to think of it, yeah, *you* should be thinking out of the left side of your brain—that's whenever you actually decide to *think*! This is just another example of you not knowing what you're talking about. I've studied this stuff, and I know what I'm saying here. Johnny needs to learn how to write with his left hand."

Mom won, as usual, and thus began my adventures of learning to become left-handed. Of course, I couldn't just teach myself, Mom said. Instead, I needed to spend the summer up East at a special boarding school where they would work with me. As an added bonus, summer school would be in session. Since I was an idiot, I could take a couple more courses there and be ready for the fall semester when—get this—I'd have to take those same, exact courses over again. If you're confused by all of this, think of what was going on in *my* mind (and I wasn't even sure if it was the left side or right side of my brain doing the processing).

Next thing I knew, Mom, Dad, and I were all on a plane to Boston. I was pretty upset; school courses and having my right hand become useless hadn't been in my summer plans. But Mom promised me that if I gave the school a look and talked to some psychologist up there, and I still didn't want to go, then she would drop the whole thing and let me live the rest of my life thinking right, *er, wrong*. My father, however, was in no mood to fly all of us up to Boston, spend the night in an expensive hotel, and then have it all be for naught. Unbeknownst to me, in his mind, I was enrolled in this program the second we got on the plane.

We took a taxi directly from the airport in Boston to some medical building downtown. Mom said I would be talking with a psychologist. I remember us sitting in a tiny waiting room, just the folks and me. I was becoming somewhat anxious, so I asked my mother what she thought the psychologist and I would be talking about.

"Johnny, remember why we're here?"

"Yeah. It's because I am thinking with my right brain instead of my left. But, at least I'm *thinking*! Dad always tells me to think—and that I'm *not* thinking! You say I *am* thinking but with the wrong side of my brain. I still don't understand how this is going to help me in school. And I can't think of one of my friends who have done something like this. Am I the only kid in the world who is thinking out of the wrong side of his brain?"

"Your friends? Well, I can't worry about them. I would bet that several of them are thinking with the wrong side of their brains, too. They just don't know it. You're lucky to have a mother who reads about this stuff and cares enough about you to spend the time and money to get help for you."

With that, the door to the waiting room swung open and in stepped the psychologist. "Johnny! Come on in! Mr. Shuchart, Mrs. Shuchart—we'll be about an hour, so if you'd like to step out and get a bite to eat or a drink, feel free to do so."

The guy walked me down the hall to an office that had a desk and a couple of chairs in it. I assumed we'd sit and talk for an hour, but the first thing he did was tell me to take off my clothes—that he needed to give me an "examination." Being eleven years old, I did what he told me, never thinking about how weird this was, that a guy who was going to evaluate me for a right brain, left brain problem needed me to strip down to my birthday suit. I must have passed the physical, because after telling me to put my clothes back on, he walked me back to the small waiting room. My parents were there, probably back from downing a few and screaming at each other about whether or not this was the dumbest thing my mother had ever done (it was). The guy who had asked me to disrobe (a pedophile, perhaps?) then took my parents away while I sat alone trying to entertain myself (iPads hadn't been invented yet). After just a few minutes my parents came back and told me we were done, that we were going out to grab some dinner.

No one said much on the elevator, or during the cab ride to some restaurant the psychologist must have suggested to my parents. After we were seated at the restaurant, my mother finally started the conversation.

"Well, Johnny, what did you think of the psychologist? What did you two talk about?"

"Not much," I said, as I played with my fork and spoon. "He just had me take my clothes off, listened to my chest, and stuff like that."

"He didn't talk to you about school, how you were doing? Huh. I can't believe that's all you did while you were in there with him. I had hoped he'd talk with you about school, your grades, and stuff like that. You're sure you didn't talk about that with him?"

"Yep, I'm sure."

"Oh, *great!*" exclaimed my father. "Jeanne, what is going on here? The guy made Johnny strip! He's a psychologist, for

God's sake! What's he doing giving our kid a physical? This is absolutely crazy!"

"Now, just wait a minute Al," interrupted Mom. "I'm sure there's a reason for what he did. He's a professional. You know, you talked to him. Frankly, I was very impressed! The man knows what he's talking about."

I was getting antsy and hungry. As I looked over the menu trying to find something to eat, my folks continued to argue. My mother wasn't backing down; she had a lot at stake, like the cost of this silly adventure. For my dad, this trip was just one more inconvenience and expense his wife and kid had caused him. He was getting angrier and angrier when the waitress showed up and took his drink order: a double Manhattan. My mom, at that point in her life, didn't drink much, but she did that night. Vodka and orange juice, I think she ordered. So there I was, sitting in a restaurant in Boston, watching my parents argue and tip a few too many, and wondering whether I should just go ahead and start my new life as a left-hander and pick up my fork with my weaker hand whenever my food arrived.

After dinner, we checked into our hotel, and all hell broke loose. I guess it was my fault, because my mother yet again asked me what I thought, and I said I wasn't going to go to this summer school—that I was okay with being right-handed (as is about 90 percent of the rest of the world).

"You *are* going to this place this summer!" screamed Dad. "I haven't been dragged up here for nothing. That's all there is to it, mister. You *will* be coming here and that's it!"

I looked at my mother and reminded her what she had promised me—that if I didn't like what I saw, I would have veto power. I guess the old man had gotten to her, because she just shook her head and told me to listen to my father. I was going and that was it.

The next day, after a long night of crying, my parents and I went to visit the place where I would soon be turned inside out. It was your typical East Coast boarding school . . . mess hall, dorms, a couple of tennis courts, definitely nothing to get excited about. We met with the headmaster, a nice old guy who consistently called me Jeffrey. (I wondered how this guy got to be the head honcho if he couldn't even remember my name.) He took us on a tour of the place. For some reason, the dorm I'd be staying in was the girls' dorm during the winter but the guys' place for summer school. (They kept the boys pretty far away from the girls, and after being there a few days I discovered why: the girls were, well, girls!).

We went back to the headmaster's office where my father signed some papers. The next thing I knew, the guy was shaking my hand and telling me how excited he was that I would be attending his fine institution. I have never forgotten the sinking feeling I had in my stomach as we got into our taxi and made our way to the airport and eventually home.

It wasn't long before I was flying back east to begin my transformation into a right-brained, left-handed young man. My parents walked me onto the plane (terrorism hadn't been invented yet, so there was no need for metal detectors) and told me to hang on to my ticket—that I was going to change planes in Baltimore and I would need it to get on the plane to Boston. Huh? So there I was: on a plane alone for the first time, and told I have to "change planes" so I can arrive at a destination I have no desire to go to. Talk about traumatic!

Somehow I made the connection in Baltimore, arrived in Boston, and was greeted by some guy, claiming to be with the school, who said he was taking me there in his car. He could have been from Mars for all I knew (I wondered if he needed an extra fishbowl to put on his head so he could breathe there). We arrived at the school late at night. My chauffer lugged my huge chest into the dorm's big common room. There I met my house parent, a nice man from Boston whose wife also worked at the school in the same job, but for the girls. My driver left and my new friend took me to my room. It had a pole standing right in the middle of it. The result was that a small room became much smaller. To make matters worse, my house parent told me my roommate had decided not to attend at the last minute (why couldn't I have *his* parents?) and that I would be the only student living alone. Could things get any worse? I remember not bothering to unpack that night. I just sat on my bed and cried.

Things not only could get worse, they did, starting as soon as I woke up the next morning. I got up, took a couple of steps, and *bang!*—I bounced off the pole and fell back onto my bed. Rubbing the new welt on the side of my face, I looked around. The room looked even smaller than it had the night before. I opened my trunk, shook my head at the amount of clothes my mother had packed, and dug out an outfit for the day. I couldn't find my toothpaste. I started tearing the trunk apart, throwing clothes everywhere like you see them do in the movies. I was crying again. I couldn't believe she forgot to give me toothpaste! I was already so angry with her for getting me into this mess, and now *this*! I flung open my door and went looking for somebody, *anybody*, from whom I could bum some toothpaste. My luck, I must have overslept. The dorm was deserted. I started yelling and screaming and running around, and still there was nobody! I dashed out the front door, expecting to see guys walking to class or beating each other up or whatever, but again . . . no one. Maybe my brain was playing tricks on me. Maybe I was just thinking with the wrong side of it again. I walked back into my room, careful this time to avoid crashing into Herman (I decided to name the pole after my never-to-appear room-mate). I sat down on my bed, looked around the clothes-strewn room, and suddenly remembered that my toothpaste was in my bathroom, right where I'd put it after I brushed my teeth the night before. I paused and then decided that my mother was still on the hook for my misery, toothpaste or not.

I finally made the move to get out of my pajamas, grab a shower, and find someplace to get something to eat. I was starving! As I was walking toward my door, it suddenly opened and there stood this short, fat, Irish-looking guy. He had red hair and equally red cheeks. I thought he must have just run a couple of miles or was having a heart attack. It turns out neither was true; he was just a roly-poly Bostonian with one of those "pahk the cah in Hahvuhd Yahd" accents.

"Hey, there, sport! How yah doing? Yah wanna go get something to eat? I'm Earl! I'm gonna be wharkin with yah this summah."

"I'm John. Can you say some of that again? I didn't quite understand what you said."

"Ah, sahree, John. Yah hungry? Let's go eat something, okay?"

Earl led the way out of the dorm and down a dirt path to the dining hall. We walked inside and, once again, found nobody. The place was empty except for us. No waiters, no busboys, nothing.

"Hey, Earl, where is everybody? I haven't seen anyone since I've been here. Am I the only kid here this summer?"

"Ah, no, there are lots of kids. They're just all in class, that's all. Yah know this is a summah school, right? Well, everybody is studying—yah know, in class. Everybody except you, that is. You're special, yah know!"

"What do you mean I'm special?"

"Hey, grab a bowl. There's some cereal ovah there. Grape Nuts, I think. Help yahself. Hmmm…looks like we're out of milk. No big deal, we'll eat the stuff with our hands! Ha!"

"Earl, you didn't tell me why I'm special."

"Oh, well you and me are gonna be wharkin on makin' you left-handed, whenever you're not in class, of course. It has something to do with your right brain, left brain problem. I'm sure they told yah all about it."

"Yeah, that's what my mom thinks. That's why she sent me here. But I figured everyone here would have that problem. You mean I'm the only one? I'm the only one who is going to learn how to become left-handed?" Now I was getting upset, and angry.

"You're the only one they've told me about," Earl sputtered, his mouth full of Grape Nuts. "So looks like it's just you and me, kid. Don't be so glum! We'll have some fun together, I promise. Hey, tell me—can you play tennis?"

"Tennis? Sure, in fact I'm a pretty decent player. Why do you want to know?"

"That's great! We have a big tournament every summah and if you're pretty good, I've got news for yah. You're gonna win! Yah use your backhand a lot?"

"No more than I have to, I guess." I had no clue what he was getting at.

"When I get through with yah, the word 'backhand' won't even be in your vocabulary any more! Yah see, you'll be using two hands from now on when you play, and they'll both be forehands! You hit a forehand shot with your right hand, and you just flip the racket ovah to your left and smash what would have been a backhand shot but is now a forehand shot! You'll kill everybody! Hurry up and finish your cereal. We gotta get stahted."

And thus began the most unbelievable eight weeks of my life. Every morning I met Earl by the tennis courts where he would have me throw a tennis ball against the backboard for thirty minutes—left-handed, of course. The first few times were a joke. I'd throw the ball as hard as I could, but sometimes it wouldn't even make it to the backboard. And when I was able to throw it the whole way, I rarely caught it as it bounced back under me, past me, or over me. I felt like an idiot chasing around after the errant tennis ball. Then, after all that, Earl would hand me a tennis racket and tell me to stand at the net.

The next hour would be excruciating. I'd stand at the net while Earl hit me ball after ball, first to my right and then to my left. Whenever he hit a shot to my left, I was supposed to flip the racket from my right hand to my left and hit the ball back over the net. I can't tell you how many balls I totally whiffed on. And whenever I got lucky and actually put the racket on the ball, the racket would go flying out of my hand. My left hand was so weak that I couldn't hold on tight enough to return the slams Earl was hitting my way. I'd get so frustrated I'd eventually throw the racket at the net and scream at Earl that I was done, that this was crazy, and that I wasn't going to do anything with my left hand…anything!

This went on for days. Same routine. After shouting that I was through, we'd pick up the rackets and balls, and Earl would walk me to my classes (summer school, remember?). I'd finally be with other kids, but most of them were older than me and seemed to know each other, so I didn't have anybody to talk with (making this wonderful experience that much more unsettling). My classes were Physics and English. What a joke! My Physics teacher looked just like Stephen Hawking (without the wheelchair) and must have been just as brilliant, because I couldn't understand anything he said. After a few days I finally got some kid to talk with me and found out it was a high school class! What was I doing here? Could the summer possibly get any worse?

Of course it could. Eventually, Earl confined my use of my right hand to when I slept. Everything, and I mean *everything* I did had to be left-handed. To ensure that I didn't sneak around and try to eat or do some other evil thing with my right hand, Earl decided to restrain my arm at times. He put it in a backward sling so it was pinned behind my back. It doesn't take a psychologist to figure out how traumatic that was for me.

After about three weeks or so, things got better. I was beginning to get the hang of playing tennis without a backhand. And school? Well, everything I did in class simply justified my parents' low opinions of my scholastic abilities. I struggled in Physics to the point where the Stephen Hawking look-alike took me aside and told me I didn't have to bother to show up in class any more; it was wasting his time as well as mine. English wasn't going much better.

By the time summer came to a close I was able to: (1) write better with my left hand than my right; (2) play tennis without ever using a backhand; (3) flunk both my school courses; and (4) wipe my rear with my left hand (no small feat). I had accomplished a lot, or so I thought until I'd been back home for a couple of weeks.

A few days into the new school year, I came home and saw my mother sitting at our breakfast room table (where she spent most of her time) reading a letter. Her sunglasses were off, which was never a good sign. She always wore them, even in the house, but took them off whenever she was angry or upset. I could tell she wasn't happy. I decided to ignore her as I opened the fridge, but she stopped me.

"I'm reading your report from summer school. We wasted a lot of money. You flunked English."

"Physics, too," I proudly interrupted.

"I can't believe you! You came back home writing and throwing and whatever with your left hand, but you flunked English! It obviously doesn't matter which side of your brain does the thinking, does it?

With that, Mom put the letter down, picked up her glass (filled with vodka, no doubt), and took a couple of sizable swigs. I decided to forgo my snack and get the heck out of the kitchen before I became even dumber than she already thought I was. Of course, I closed the fridge with my left hand, thanks to her!

Reframing Becoming Ambidextrous

I still remember how lonely and scared I was during the first days of the summer school. I had that sinking feeling in the pit of my stomach that we all have felt at one time or another—a feeling that has only recently receded when I think back on this event. For many years I've struggled with the impact that summer had on me. How could my parents have put me under such stress? Didn't they think about the trauma I'd be going through—from standing naked in front of some child psychiatrist to hopping a plane alone to having my good hand literally pinned behind my back? And after all of that, I still hadn't improved mentally. Nothing had changed. If I'd had a right brain, left brain problem at the *start* of the summer, I had one at the end—and probably still do!

There is one saving grace in all of this. Whenever I tell this story, it never fails to get big laughs. And, as I've said, whenever you make people laugh, it's hard not to laugh with them. So, a couple of things have helped me reframe this incredible experience: (1) my sense of humor has allowed me to "laugh it off" and release the trauma from this adventure; and (2) I've realized that learning to use my left hand was one of the most useful things I've ever done! After a total of seventeen operations in the past fifteen years, many on my right shoulder and right wrist, I've never missed a beat—not to mention still being able to wipe my behind with either hand!

Chapter 5

"Get a date? Are you kidding me?"

"Pretty much everyone hates high school. It's a measure of your humanity, I suspect. If you enjoyed high school, you were probably a psychopath or a cheerleader. Or possibly both."
—Jenny Lawsen

My high school career, as I reflect upon it, didn't really start until after the tenth grade. That's when I switched schools. Up until that time, I'd been attending an all-boys private school. (If you recall, this is the school that accepted me after I flunked the entrance exam only because my brother, the Genius, was already a student, and the school probably needed someone to bring down its grade point average to avoid accusations of grade creep.) I had fought my parents to leave that school from the first day when they made us play football. I was into baseball and basketball as a kid, but had never put on shoulder pads in my life. I remember that after lunch on the first day of school, they had us kids schlep over to the gym where they assigned us each a locker. Then we lined up at the school's athletic store, an obvious profit source along with the pay phone just inside the front door. We had to sign the bill for gold pants, a red jersey, a white helmet, white socks, shoes with plastic cleats, and something I had never, ever seen before: a jock strap.

I lugged all this equipment back to my locker where I sat down and wondered what I was supposed to do next. Beyond putting on the socks I was lost. The pants had pockets all over them—on the thighs, the knees, the tailbone, everywhere. Attached to them was a plastic bag full of things that looked like sponges. (I learned later that these were pads, which you put into the pant's pockets. They were designed to deflect the blow from the fat guy squatting across from you on the field who was told to kill you as soon as he heard "hike!") Fortunately, there was a student whose locker wasn't far from mine who seemed to know what he was doing, so whenever he wasn't looking, I would steal a glance to see how he was putting on all of these items. It took me forever to get dressed; in fact, I was the last one out onto the field. I think I'd still be at my locker if I hadn't given up entirely on the jock strap. I had no clue what to do with it and there was no way I was going to get caught peeking at this other kid while he was putting his on.

After we all gathered on the field, the coach lined us up and told each of us to "go out for a pass." Since I was the last in line I had a chance to figure out what that meant, sort of. Our class had sixty-some fifth graders and, from what I could tell, only a couple of us had a clue as to what to do. Most of the kids ran around in circles with their arms up in the air while the coach screamed at them to run in a straight line. It didn't seem to matter; the only throws the kids caught were the ones that hit them in the head and fell into their hands.

When my turn came I was determined to do it correctly. So I did; I ran in a straight line for about three feet and stopped. Of course I, too, put my arms up in the air and the ball went right through them. That was as close as I ever came to catching a football that year.

I bring up this incident because, for some reason, it has stuck with me all these years. I don't know if it was the embarrassment of not knowing what to do with the jock strap, of looking like a klutz trying to make my first-ever catch, or of taking a communal shower after practice and seeing my first uncircumcised penis (wow, was that a shock!). Whatever it was, I think I knew from that day on that I wanted to go to a school where I didn't have to flunk the entrance exam to get in.

Eventually, my parents relented and let me transfer to a public school. It helped that brother Steve had pulled rank and transferred after his tenth grade, too. His reasons for wanting out were different from mine though. His grades were great, the teachers loved him, and he was a superstar on the golf team, but he had fallen in love, and she went to the local public high school. I think Steve had figured out that he was smart enough to get into any college he wanted, so where he attended school didn't much matter. (He ended up graduating with straight A's and enrolling in Tulane because the food in New Orleans was incredible and the drinking age was eighteen—not to mention that it was pretty easy to buy motorcycles there, as you'll read later.) My reasons for wanting to switch schools were long in the making (think jock straps), and though they had nothing to do with girls initially, someone special did come into my life over the summer. And had I not transferred schools, my children might not be redheaded, smart, or good-looking—all attributes that everyone will confirm are the direct result of my wife's great genes and abilities.

My first date with my future wife, Stevie, was a very awkward and uncomfortable experience. Ironically, we had known each other since we were both four years old while attending preschool together. But my family became rich (or so it seemed at the time), and we moved up a couple of social notches, which required us to also improve our residential address. Moving away meant changing schools, so I hadn't seen Stevie for years when we ran into each other while attending the same Jewish confirmation class after tenth grade. As luck would have it, I hitched a ride with a friend whose girlfriend was sleeping over at Stevie's, and the four of us ended up going out for ice cream after class. I had no clue how to act; I'd had one date in my life, and that had been a bust. Fortunately, the two lovebirds in our midst kept us entertained, so I didn't have to say much. It turned out to be no big deal, and I didn't think anything about it until my phone rang a couple of weeks later.

On the other end of the call was my brother's girlfriend. She told me she had four tickets to the St. Louis Cardinals' baseball game for that night and that I should get a date and join the two of them. I remember laughing, declining as quickly as possible, reminding her that I had nobody to call and didn't want to call anybody even if I had, but told her I'd love to go if I could bring with me anyone or anything other than a girl. She replied that I needed to tell my date to be ready at 7:15 p.m. She added that if I couldn't find a date, she'd find one for me, and she was sure I'd like my own choice a lot better than hers. She then hung up.

I felt trapped and a little sick to my stomach. I opened my desk drawer to find my little "black book" of hot numbers. Instead, I came up with a brown book containing a couple of pieces of torn blank paper. I thought, "Who do I know?" That took less than a second to answer…nobody! My mother was home so I went into the kitchen to see if she could help.

"Mom, I need a date."

"Oh, I didn't know you liked dates. I'll put them on the grocery list."

"Uh, no, I need a real date, with a girl. And I need one for tonight."

"You're kidding!" Mom laughed. "*You* want to get a date… and for tonight?"

"Look, it isn't my idea. Can you help me out? Do you know somebody who has a kid that I can take to the ball game, somebody's daughter who likes baseball and knows how to act on a date?"

"No! And you don't, either. Don't be ridiculous. Now leave me alone, can't you see I'm on the phone?"

Of course, Mom was always on the phone, which never stopped any of us from talking to her, nor her from carrying on a conversation with us and with whoever was on the other end of the line. I walked back to my room and began thinking about which illness would soon be striking me. Steve and his girlfriend wouldn't want to be with someone carrying a serious, communicable disease, right? Maybe malaria or typhoid? With no Internet (another thing that hadn't been invented yet) at my disposal, I wasn't able to research the symptoms I should be displaying, so I began making them up. A high fever is always a good thing to have, along with red splotches, if you want to keep others at bay. I'll also throw in some coughing and wheezing—easy things to fake.

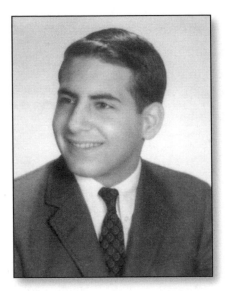

Age 16. No wonder Stevie fell for me!

Just then, Steve walked into the house and straight into my room, which usually only happened when he either wanted money or needed for me to put his bedroom window screens back into place after he snuck out of the house. No such luck this time.

"Hey, kid! I hear you're getting a date for tonight! Who's the unlucky gal?"

Steve had appeared too quickly. I hadn't had time to put on my Southeast Asian soon-to-be-terminal disease act. His entrance startled me into another one of my stupid, clumsy moments.

"Uh, Stevie. I asked Stevie to go with me."

"Stevie? Wait, is that the little kid we went to school with back in the Moorlands? Last time I saw her she didn't have any teeth. And really curly hair. Is that who we're talking about?"

"She has teeth now, and I think her hair grew out, or she bought an iron to straighten it or something."

"Well, I'm glad you got somebody, kid. I'm really looking forward to tonight. You're taking a big step. Hey, you think you'll kiss her goodnight?"

If he only knew that at the moment the only thing I'd be kissing would be my hand. I hadn't even called her yet! What was I going to do if she didn't want to go with me (a very real possibility) . . . lie and say that *she* was the one who suddenly came down with malaria?

I was screwed. I looked at the clock; it was already 3:00 p.m. She'd probably already made plans for the night anyway. I snuck into my brother's room when he was in the kitchen and found his school telephone directory (Stevie went to the same school he had transferred to). I called Stevie's number, and her sister answered and said she wasn't home, that she was at work (she volunteered at a hospital). I asked if she knew whether or not Stevie was busy that night and was told "maybe." I asked how I could get in touch with her, and she said she doubted she could reach her, but that she would try to leave her a message to call home in the next hour or so (girls didn't ever call guys back then . . . ever!).

Turns out Stevie and I were able to connect and, before I knew it, I was ringing her front doorbell, more than half-hoping I was at the wrong house and I could go to the game alone. As I was just about to start my retreat from the front steps, the door flung open and there stood Stevie's father. He looked just like I remembered him from when I was in the second grade: hair straight back, big smile, and short— very short. He was warm and friendly, extending his hand and inviting me in. I walked past their living room and into the family room where I was stunned to be confronted by a welcoming committee consisting of Stevie's mother, grand-father, sister, and an aunt and uncle visiting from out of town. Scared to death, standing there in my madras shirt and black khakis, I turned just in time to see Stevie come walking out from her room. She was dressed to the nines! I thought, "This isn't going to turn out very well,"—me in khakis, her in high heels and a dress. This was an omen, however: we have spent more than fifty years together, and we rarely dress like we're going to the same places together.

I fumbled my way through some introductions and then promptly headed out the front door, Stevie trailing about two steps behind me (remember, I had no clue how to act with a girl). We hopped into the car, and I could see my brother and his girlfriend smiling as if they had just helped to pull off the biggest coup of the year (forcing me to get a date). I remember thinking that if I was going to die some time in the near future, this would be as good a time as any, sparing me from what I feared was going to be the worst three hours of my life.

Boy, was I wrong. I should have died at the *end* of the three hours. It was only the worst *ending* of a night I had ever lived through! Not because of anything Stevie did; in fact, she was fun the whole evening. Her knowledge of baseball equaled my knowledge of Einstein's theory of relativity, so we avoided talking about either, but we did spend lots of time laughing and reminiscing about our early grade school experiences together. Everything was going great...until it was time to take her home.

I wasn't old enough to drive yet so after we went to a party at some guy's house after the baseball game, I needed my brother's help to schlep Stevie home. He was busy downing a few brews, so he asked a friend of his to do it.

I forgot to mention that the St. Louis Cardinals had won the National League pennant in 1964, so at every home game in 1965 they gave out souvenir World Series drinking glasses. Since none of the rest of us wanted them, we each gave ours to Stevie (not that she wanted them, either). So that night, as we got out of the car at her house, Stevie was fumbling with her purse and four glasses. To this day, I swear this is what happened: she got out of the car, turned to me, and said, "thank you, and goodnight!" I assumed that meant "goodnight, John," so I said "you're welcome" and stood at the car as I watched her walk to her front door, juggling four glasses as she frantically looked through her purse to find her house key. Of course, I didn't move to rescue her . . . after all, she had told me "goodnight"! I'd just assumed she must not have wanted me to walk her to her door. To this day I don't know how she managed to get her key out of her purse and into the lock without dropping those glasses.

I got back into the car and my brother's friend just stared at me. "You idiot! What are you doing? Why didn't you walk her to the door?" I told him she said "goodnight" to me at the car!

"No! She told *me* goodnight, not *you!*" He then became the worst prognosticator ever when he said, "Well, you really blew that one . . . you'll never see her again."

More than fifty years later, every one of my days ends with her telling me "goodnight."

Reframing My Incredibly Rude Behavior on My Big Date

Going on your first or second real date can be (and was) very stressful, to say the least, especially when you've gone to an all-boys school for six years straight. I had no idea how to act around girls. What was I supposed to talk about—clothes or something? It was tough enough as a teenager to talk to *anybody*!

But I think my date with Stevie went more smoothly than I ever anticipated because we did find something to talk about: our past. We laughed about our first and second grade teachers and remembered some funny things that happened during Christmas season at school. The population of our elementary school was about 90 percent Jewish, but that didn't stop the school from buying a huge Christmas tree that greeted us each year in the middle of the front forum. It also didn't stop our teachers from having us sing innumerable Christmas carols, even though we didn't know most of the words. I remember a student asking why we never sang Chanukah songs. The teacher said that would be no problem at all—in fact, it was a great idea. She asked the kid to sing one and he didn't know any. That took care of that, no Chanukah songs for us!

The ending to that first date is something we've argued about for years. Did Stevie turn to me or to the driver and say, "thank you, goodnight"? *She* maintains that only an idiot (me) would think she had wanted to walk to her door alone holding four very breakable drinking glasses while also carrying a purse and having to dig out her house key. I, however, am positive she was as nervous as I was and would have done anything to keep me from kissing her goodnight.

Fifty years later, I still don't know for sure what happened, but I've felt embarrassed for how I let that night end. I think I was so preoccupied with what my brother had said ("Hey, you think you'll kiss her good-night?") that my mind went totally blank when Stevie and I got out of the car. Not walking her to the door ranks right up there with many of the other really dumb, embarrassing things I've done in my life. We all do some things we regret, and we can't understand why we did them, but we need to learn to let them go—chalk them up to something and move on. And when you mess up with a woman, it probably helps if you end up marrying her!

Chapter 6

"You are not the brightest of my four sons."

"I have never let my schooling interfere with my education."
—Mark Twain

It started to become clear that my right brain, left brain "problem" either had never existed or was never resolved, because my grades in middle and high school seldom rose above a C+. I had a decent year or two, but getting top grades wasn't an everyday occurrence. I remember once getting a B on some small project and my parents taking me out to dinner to celebrate!

My mother's frustration with me reached a boiling point during my senior year in high school. My English teacher wrote her a personal note saying that my skills were so poor I would never pass freshman English in college, regardless of what school I might attend ("not that Johnny would be accepted anywhere"). He said that my parents would be wasting their money on any further education for me and that their best hope was that I might one day obtain a skill that I could use to earn a living—you know, something like cleaning up after a horse parade.

To this day, I have no idea what prompted this dorky, weasel-looking teacher to write that note. He had taught my brother the year before, and since Steve wrote poetry and prose like Walt Whitman or somebody, this guy just loved him. Being only a year behind Steve, I always got his teachers right after he had them, and they expected me to also be a genius. When it became evident that I wasn't, some of them had trouble accepting it. *They also kept forgetting I had a right brain, left brain problem!*

My mother certainly remembered, and that's what made this teacher's note so devastating. After all, she had paid to have me turned into a lefty in the hopes that it would rewire my brain. I think, up until this point, she had held out hope that all the effort and money she'd spent on overhauling me would pay off in spite of my poor showing in the English course I took that infamous summer. My high school English teacher's comments said otherwise.

In spite of being told I would never be accepted into a college and that I would flunk out even if I were, I applied to three schools: the University of Colorado, the University of Wisconsin, and Tulane University. I liked the idea of Colorado since the legal age for consuming 3.2 percent alcohol beer was eighteen, and also I'd learn how to snow ski. Wisconsin was somewhat familiar to me since I had gone to camp in Madison in third or fourth grade. Tulane was a no-brainer; Steve was there, so it had to be a fun place, and he could show me the dopes, er, ropes.

My mother knew, of course, that I had applied to these colleges since there was a small application fee for each and she had to pay them (my ten-dollars-a-week allowance was for more important things). However, she had never been confident that I was looking at the right schools, which is probably what prompted her to stop into my room one Saturday afternoon. I was lying on my bed watching a football game on TV when she arrived. It was 1966 and Michigan State and Notre Dame were playing. At the time, the two teams were ranked as the two best, so it was a huge game, with the winner most likely to be crowned the National Champion. When Mom came in to see me, I knew the game wasn't going to be the subject of her visit, but I was hoping that whatever she had to say would be brief enough so I could keep watching.

"You know," she began, "I've been doing some thinking, and since you are not the brightest of my four sons, I'm pretty sure you're not going to get accepted by any of those three schools you've applied to." With that, she turned and glanced at the television.

"Who is playing?"

"Michigan State and Notre Dame," I snapped.

"Well," she said, "Notre Dame is out, of course (we're Jewish!)—I want you to apply to Michigan State." With that, she turned and walked out of my room.

Apply to Michigan State? Was she serious? I couldn't believe what I had just heard! But if it sounded bizarre then, about ten days later it *really* blew my mind when she asked me if I'd received the application yet (remember, no email or faxes back then, just snail mail).

"No, I didn't write for one. I'm not going to Michigan State. I'm going to one of the schools I've already applied to."

"Listen! You are *not* getting into those schools! You will be lucky to get into *any* school! You read what your English teacher wrote. You know you have a right brain, left brain problem. You know you're not the brightest kid I have. Now send for the application to Michigan State and do it *now*! I have a friend whose daughter goes there and she loves it." (That meant to me that her friend's kid must also be an idiot and unable to get into a college anywhere else other than good old MSU.)

I was crushed. I mean, was I really the dumbest kid in the family? Okay, Steve had me, but by now I had two much younger brothers, not yet six and four years old, and was Mom telling me she already knew they were brighter than me? Was she right? Was I doomed to attend a trade school and maybe learn how to change a flat tire or peel oranges or something? Well, not quite. It turns out I was accepted at Colorado *and* Tulane and was wait-listed at Wisconsin. And, after all that, I actually did end up attending Michigan State, not because I had to, but because, by that time, I wanted to. I'd learned that Michigan State had started a really exciting immersion program in the Russian language, which was an interest of mine (I thought at one time I wanted to join the CIA, but when I learned they shoot at you when you're an agent, I decided against it). There was also another reason I went to Michigan State. Though it wasn't exactly my idea, Wisconsin was ruled out—even had the university ended up accepting me.

By that time, I was going steady with Stevie, my future wife. Her parents had known my folks for years. (Remember, we had all lived in the Moorlands in Clayton, Missouri, and Stevie and I walked to the same elementary school every day.) But, just because our parents knew each other didn't mean they *liked* each other. In fact, the opposite was true: they had absolutely no love lost between them. That really didn't surprise me. My folks were, well, my folks. Stevie's parents were warm, social, and supportive of their kids; they shared a loving marriage and enjoyed being with extended family. If it sounds like oil and water getting together, that's exactly what it was. Our two families never socialized throughout the entire time Stevie and I dated, except for one fateful evening. I don't know exactly how it happened or who initiated it, but our parents decided to meet at Stevie's house for a night of bridge playing . . . or so we were told.

Bridge turned out to be an excuse for the four of them to discuss Stevie and me and our relationship. It was, I discovered later, my parents' objective to persuade my future in-laws that Stevie and I should not be allowed to attend the same college (assuming I ever got into one, of course). My parents didn't like anyone on the other side of the table, neither of Stevie's parents nor Stevie herself, and they were determined to do whatever they could to ensure that they would never have to consider them family. They assumed if Stevie and I went to different schools that at least one of us would find someone else to marry. My parents won, and we ended up being forced to attend different schools for at least our first year.

Stevie could have attended just about any school in the country. She finished seventh in our high school class of over 400 (which *did* include me!), aced her SATs, and submitted dynamite college applications. But, love won out, and since I'd decided upon East Lansing, Michigan, Stevie narrowed her choices to the best schools closest by. Ironically, she wound up attending Wisconsin, the one school where I failed to get accepted.

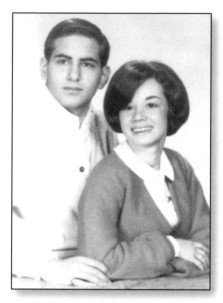

Going steady in high school

Going to different schools affected our future only by lowering our net worth. Stevie and I had both worked the summer before college and together saved over 800 dollars, a huge sum in 1967. We ended up using every penny during the school year on phone calls, airplanes, trains, buses, and motels (back then the phone calls alone cost nearly 3 dollars to place a three-minute call). We saw each other at least every six weeks. And after our freshman year, Stevie transferred to Michigan State. In spite of the fact that each of us *did* date other people and had some major issues come up, fifty years later we have two super kids and two adorable grandchildren. Sending us to different schools was obviously a failed (and expensive) exercise by our parents.

Reframing Being Rejected by My Parents and a Rogue Teacher

I still can't believe the gall of my English teacher! In my day it wasn't unusual for report cards to be accompanied by written comments from teachers; in fact it was expected. But it was virtually unheard of for a teacher to send a personal note to a student's home. I'm guessing the school knew nothing about it and that a copy was never included in my file. It absolutely should never have been written.

Maybe English wasn't my best subject back then, but in retrospect, just how dumb could I have been if I could learn Russian? I began studying it in eighth grade, and by my senior year in high school I could speak it almost fluently. Why didn't my parents ever give me credit for *that*? To this day, whenever I speak Russian or someone finds out I know the language they're in awe. "Wow, Russian! You must be smart!" Little do they know!

I don't have to tell you that words can hurt and can cause severe, long-lasting trauma, especially when they come from our parents. It doesn't take a psychiatrist to figure that out. And when my mother essentially told me that I was a loser—that I'd never be acceptable to her, that she wasn't proud of me, and that I wasn't "the brightest of her four sons"—well, it was pretty painful.

Thankfully, my experience as an educator has taught me that grades aren't the only gauge of a kid's intelligence or potential. When I look back upon my English teacher's note to my parents and their continual reminder to me that I wasn't their brightest son, I can't help but think of how wrong I've proven them. Just think: if my English is really so poor, how can I possibly write a book? If I'm not smart enough to get into a college, how did I end up graduating from Michigan State with honors? If I was such a loser, why was I elected president of my fraternity? And why would the *Kansas City Business Journal* write articles about my successes and label me as a "Serial Entrepreneur" and a "hometown hero?"

I've learned to laugh at how things have turned out; I'm the failure who didn't fail, and that fact helps me to manage the terribly painful trauma caused me by the many words my parents and others said about my intelligence and potential to become a success.

My mother spent a lot of time reminding me how dumb I was. My father's turn to up the ante is coming up next….

Chapter 7
Grounded 90 days and out 250 bucks!

"Never learn to do anything; if you don't learn,
you'll always find someone else to do it for you."
—Mark Twain

My brother was the epitome of this quote from Mark Twain. He *always* had someone else—me!—doing things for him, especially his dirty work.

The best example of Steve's ability to put me *in* harm's way and him *out* of it occurred during his freshman year at Tulane University in New Orleans. It all started when he came home for his Christmas break. One of the first things he said to me when he got home was, "I need to borrow 250 dollars. I'm buying a motorcycle, and you're financing it for me."

"You're joking, right?"

"Dead serious, kid."

Considering that my father had told us on several occasions that even *riding* on a motorcycle was *verboten*, my response was pretty direct. "You can't. This time the old man will totally, completely kill you."

"Screw him. I don't care," Steve said in response. "Just give me the money. And you can't get into trouble. How's he ever gonna find out? It isn't like I'm planning on giving him a ride on it or anything. And if it's the money you're worried about, you know I'm good for it."

Spoken by a guy who never, ever paid me back. For anything. I lent him money for dates, for booze, for whatever he wanted. Pay me back? *Steve?* He couldn't pull the wallet out of his pocket with both hands!

Nevertheless, as usual, I wrote him a check, but this time I actually put it to my lips and kissed it "good-bye" as I handed it to him. So why would I give Steve the money? Money I knew I would never see again? Money that was going to purchase something Dad had always told us we couldn't ever have? ("Not while you're living under *my* roof!") I'll tell you why: because he was my brother, plain and simple. Something the old man never understood, as you'll soon read.

Well, about two weeks after I gave him the cash, Steve left for his return engagement at Tulane. I'd had a pretty decent time with him while he was home, but was ready for him to go back. He had mostly spent his time in his room eating cheese popcorn and chugging Vess Red Cream Soda, so there wasn't a whole lot of interaction between us. Nevertheless, him just being around created tension between my parents. Mother was his great protector, the old man his great antagonist, and I—well, I guess I was just his banker. Anyway, he hopped a plane back to New Orleans, and I resumed playing out the string to my high school career.

About three weeks later, I walked into my room after another typically annoying day in the life of a high school senior, threw my ridiculously heavy pile of books on my desk (backpacks hadn't been invented yet), and lay down on my bed for what I hoped was going to be a nice little snooze before dinner. No sooner had I closed my eyes than my phone rang. Since caller ID hadn't been invented yet either (what exactly *had* been invented?), I picked up the receiver, and before I could utter a word, my banking client (Steve) began talking about as fast as someone does at the end of those radio commercials where they have to tell the *truth* about their great offer in three and a half seconds.

"Hey, listen, kid...in about twenty minutes some guy is going to call you and ask if it's okay if I buy a motorcycle... and you're going to have to play like you're Dad."

"What?" I asked, half not remembering about the great motorcycle caper and half not wanting to.

He'd already hung up.

I was left holding the phone in a daze. How in the hell was I going to be my dad? Already starting to sweat, I did a three-sixty of my room. My eyes locked onto my new, *loud* electric typewriter. Ah ha! I could turn it on when this guy called, and if I stretched my arm out as much as possible, I could grab the phone receiver in my right hand while I typed with my left. The guy would think I really was my dad, working hard in an office! (And yes, I *am* the inventor of the world's first virtual office.) The only thing missing was the voice: I looked like a teenager and, worse, I *sounded* like one. My charade was missing a critical element. I decided there was nothing I could do but to try to speak in my best baritone imitation.

About twenty minutes later, just as Steve had warned, my phone rang.

"Mr. Shuchart?"

"Yes, this is Mr. Shuchart," I answered, and, with perspiration now streaming down my face, lowered my voice as far as it would go. "Mr. Shuchart here—what can I do for you?"

I felt like an idiot. I was wondering if the guy was buying my act when he asked me the big question of the day.

"I've got your son in here now and he's not eighteen years of age yet and, by law, here in New Orleans, I need your permission for him to buy this motorcycle he's looking at."

Hmmm. I'm thinking, "Doesn't he need something in writing from Dad—er, me? Perhaps a fax with my signature on it?" (Oops…faxes weren't invented yet either.) Obviously, all he wanted to do was to sell a motorcycle the fastest, most hassle-free way possible.

"Well, how's he paying for this?" I asked, trying to answer the way any father worth his fatherhood would have responded.

I heard the guy then put his hand over the receiver and ask my brother, "Your dad wants to know how you're paying for this. Is this *your* money?"

After a few seconds of muffled conversation, the guy comes back and says, "He's got his own money. Do you want to talk to him?"

"Damn right, I want to talk to him," I said, starting to really get into this fatherhood shtick.

Steve got on the phone and I just blasted him. "Dad's gonna kill us! You are out of your mind…and I'm out 250 bucks! I sure hope you have fun riding on *my* bike! You're insane— you're gonna get killed or something and then I'll never get my money back!"

Steve, ever the cool, calm, and collected one, stayed in character, and rather than arguing with me or slamming the phone down, he thanked me (Dad) for giving my permission and hung up.

I got off the phone and off my typewriter and fell into my desk chair, exhausted and confused as to what had just happened. I had helped my brother many times before, lying to my father as to his whereabouts when he was late for dinner or some other chaotic family event, or putting the screen back on his window when he escaped after hours to go see a girlfriend. But this time was different. This time I had helped him do something that we had been warned never to do by the old man. This time I had helped him purchase a 700-pound, two-wheeling machine that could kill him if he wasn't careful.

I conked out on my bed, asleep in a minute, and was awakened only by the sound of the garage door opening. I checked my watch, and I knew immediately that it was my father. He always got home at a quarter to six (remember, we lived the life of precision: "Yes, Sir! No, Sir! No excuse, Sir!"). So it wasn't a surprise to hear the garage door—and, right after, the door leading into the house—open at precisely five forty-five. What followed, though, wasn't ordinary. As soon as Dad stepped into the house, I heard him warn my mother, "Do *not* come in!"

That was it. "Do *not* come in!"

The next thing I heard was the sound of footsteps coming to my room.

Somewhat alarmed but not yet panicked, I watched as the old man opened my door, grabbed my desk chair, and swung it around Western style before plopping down on it.

"Now, you know how this works. When you tell me things I ought to know *before* I tell you that I already know them, the punishment is a lot less severe, right?"

"Right," I said, thinking, *"Oh, sh*t!* What's going on here?"

"So, do you have anything you want to tell me?"

Not being the brightest of my parents' four sons (a fact of which my mother constantly reminded me), my mind went blank. I knew Dad couldn't possibly know about the motorcycle. I mean, I'd done such a convincing job of being Mr. Shuchart. The deal was signed, sealed, and delivered. Steve was undoubtedly riding around New Orleans with some great-looking chick hanging on while I waited in my room for what was obviously going to be a discussion that would live in my personal infamy.

As I sat on my bed staring at my soon-to-be-raving father, I tried to think of something he must already have known about before I had to start this round of Jewish Confession—which, by the way, is similar to what the Catholics do except Catholics get forgiven, while we Jews never do. (My parents remember everything I've ever done to shun their love and adoration and, well, once scarred, they never heal.) Since I had no clue as to what the old man could have possibly discovered, I started telling him things from my earliest memories—reciting the entire encyclopedia of everything I'd ever done wrong.

He listened to each and every tale of woe, nodding along, never changing expression or his position in my chair.

Each time I incriminated myself, he would ask if there was something else coming his way.

I'd pause and, thinking lots of information would be better than a little, continue with, "Yeah, there was that time I helped Steve get out of the...."

Finally, after about thirty minutes, he asked if I was finished—if I had anything else he needed to know.

"I'm done," I sighed. Again, the motorcycle thing never entered my mind, because it was impossible that he could have known about it. Absolutely *impossible*! My only worry was that I had spilt too much—that whatever he had on me was really minor and this had been a test to see whether or not I'd live up to his credo of "Yes, Sir! No, Sir! No excuse, Sir!"

"Are you sure you're done? There's nothing else you have to say, nothing you need to tell me?" He was giving me one, final chance to save myself. "Remember, if *I* tell *you*, the punishment will be much more severe...*much*!"

Totally exasperated, I finally asked, "What is it that you want me to *tell* you?" I mean, I had told him absolutely everything...*everything* except for the one thing he couldn't possibly know about. What on earth could he have on me that I hadn't already pleaded guilty to?

Well, little did I know, nor would I find out for years, that my dad had "secretly" opened an office in New Orleans, basically so he could keep an eye on my brother. Those monthly "out of town" trips he was taking were obviously to New Orleans. Had we had a better relationship—make that *any* kind of "normal" relationship—I would have asked where he was going and he would have told me. But, with my father, you lived under the "don't ask, don't tell" rule. Meanwhile, it turns out the motorcycle salesman had been suspicious of my pre-puberty-sounding gurgling as well as my phony electric typewriter background noise. (I guess the virtual office idea would have to wait another few years.) The salesman started hunting around and discovered that the New Orleans phone book listed one Alvin J. Shuchart. Why this greedy, do-anything-to-close-a-sale guy would do a one-eighty and become a do-gooder and protector of all parents is beyond me, but the guy called my father's listing, and even though Dad wasn't in town at the time, here again the gods were working against me. Turns out Dad had a cleaning lady (we called these people "maids" or much worse back in those days) come to his apartment once every couple of weeks, and *she decided to answer his phone*—something I am positive she wasn't supposed to do! So when the salesman asked for my father, she said he wasn't home, but that she would be happy to give him my father's St. Louis office number, which for some crazy reason he had given to her. ARGH!

Equipped with the number, the guy must now have thought he was Columbo (the trench coat–wearing, cigar–smoking, bumbling, sneaky, but extremely effective detective). I assume that when he got my old man on the phone and told him the whole story, he was probably expecting a medal or a big reward or something. I doubt he got anything but a tongue lashing from the old man for selling a bike to an underage kid.

I remember waiting nervously as the old man rested his chin on the back of my chair, tapping his fingers a few times, all the while staring at the floor. It was the first time in minutes he had moved, thus ending all hope that the stress of interrogating me had caused him to suffer a fatal heart attack. In many ways, I think these were the worst few seconds of my life, waiting to see what he was going to do. He obviously had *something* on me, but what on earth could it be? I was going nuts—so much so that it was actually a huge relief when he finally raised his head and began to speak. For a man so close to killing his own son, he was actually pretty composed and calm.

"I want you to tell me why you helped your brother buy a motorcycle."

Have you ever been caught with your hand in the cookie jar? Busted for an extramarital affair? Hidden the fact you were Bernie Madoff's right-hand man? I felt a bolt of lightning race through my body, starting around my hips and quickly migrating up to my neck. My head then exploded in pain, and I never in my life felt like puking as much as I did at that moment. I remember wishing Steve was in the room so I could kill him, but, as usual, he was nowhere to be found, leaving me to once again fend off the old man for something he had talked me into doing.

I couldn't think of anything to say, so I blurted out the first thing to come to mind, and as soon as I did, I knew I had just buried myself. "Why did I do it? Because he asked me to. Brothers do things like this for each other."

"Wrong answer!" Dad screamed. "You don't help your brother. You tell your parents!"

"But what if—"

"No buts about it."

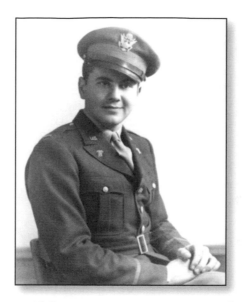

Big Al: "Yes, Sir! No, Sir! No excuse, Sir!"

And then, he lowered the boom. Standing up and putting my chair back under my desk, he looked at me, took a quick, short breath (don't nice, calm people take *long* breaths before they pass sentence?) and told me to hand over my car keys and driver's license. (If I had been sixty-five he would have probably demanded my Medicare card, too.)

"You're grounded for *at least* the next ninety days. You will go straight to and from school. You understand? You have any questions? Am I clear?"

"Um, how am I supposed to get to school, now that I don't have a car?"

THAT was definitely the wrong question. This time he went ballistic.

"How you get to school is YOUR problem. I don't care if you walk, crawl, or ride a tricycle, but you WILL go to school, you will get there ON TIME, and you will get your butt home every day by four o'clock." (I instinctively wanted to ask him if I could get a motorcycle for the commute to school just to see if it would bring on a stroke, but decided against it.)

With that he opened my door and, slamming it behind him, began ranting at my mother: "I'm gonna kill those kids, Jeanne, I'm gonna kill 'em. This is YOUR fault! Do *not* go into that room. Leave him alone and do not think for one minute you will be able to rescue him. *This* time they have gone too far. I've had it!"

If you're hoping, like I did, that this story had a happy ending—that there is some sort of justice in the world and brother Steve got what was coming to him—well, forget it.

Three weeks later to the day, Stevie (not to be confused with my dearest brother Steve) was in New Orleans checking out Sophie Newcomb College as the institute of higher learning she might attend in the fall.

She called me that night. "Guess what I did today?" she said, sounding almost giddy.

"I have no clue," I answered, never in a trillion years expecting to hear what came over the phone next.

"I rode on your motorcycle! Isn't that funny?"

"What?" Did I actually hear what I thought I heard?

"Yeah!...I was walking down the street, your brother spotted me, stopped, and gave me a ride."

"On MY motorcycle?"

"It's a pretty cool bike," she said, sounding way too excited for my tastes.

"Let me get this straight," I said. "I'm grounded for ninety days, I have no driver's license, no car, no hope of ever getting paid back my 250 dollars, and Steve's riding around with my girlfriend, having the time of his life. Are you *KIDDING* me?"

"Johnny, I'm thinking there's a disconnect here. You see, I don't think Steve thinks he did anything wrong. He just thinks you messed up the call with the sales guy. Steve said something to me about if you had done a better job playing your father, the guy would never have tried to find him and everybody would have gone home happy. I think that's why he also told me you didn't deserve your money back. I gotta tell you, Steve seems pretty happy on that bike!"

I was livid. As soon as I hung up with Stevie I raced into the kitchen and confronted my mother (the old man was out of town, looking after my brother, my girlfriend, and my motorcycle, I assumed).

Mom must have heard me on the phone with Stevie, because she was ready for me as soon as I opened my mouth.

"You did wrong and you got punished for it," she said.

"How is it reasonable to only punish me?" I asked.

"He's in college," she said by way of explanation.

"And so?"

"What do you want us to do? Call him every minute and ask his whereabouts? The best you can hope for out of all this is that you get your money back, but we both know that will never happen. You *did* kiss that check you gave him good-bye, didn't you?"

ARGH!

How I've Reframed Getting Framed

My struggles with this incident have revolved around a couple of emotions: First, I feel sorry I disappointed my parents by supporting Steve; second, I have never been sure how I *should* feel toward Steve. Should I be angry with him for even asking me to participate in his charade? Should I be upset he never got any punishment whatsoever and never paid me back my 250 bucks? Or, should I really believe what I told my father— that brothers stick up for each other and that's just the way it is?

The real villain in all of this certainly wasn't me; that honor goes to Steve. It was he who decided not to follow Dad's rules. It was he who decided to do whatever was necessary in order to procure the motorcycle. Steve set me up, plain and simple, and to this day I'm still not sure he cared about my fate. He surely knew that if anyone was going to escape unscathed, it would be him, not me. I was still living at home under the scrutiny of our parents. He was in faraway New Orleans and out of their reach. Short of taking him out of school (something Jewish parents would have a difficult time doing since it might prevent their dear child from becoming a lawyer or doctor!), there wasn't much they could do to him if we were caught.

The other part of the equation, though, is my father. For years I was more upset with him than with anyone else. He was clearly full of anger and frustration and took out his angst on me by handing down what I still consider to be an unjust sentence. But now, as a parent myself, my perspective has changed somewhat. I, too, would have been angry if my older son had disobeyed my rules. I would have also been concerned for his safety (I've always wondered if this played a bigger part in the old man's thinking than I realized; I certainly hope so). And there's no doubt I'd be upset with my other son for helping his brother do something I considered dangerous, and for lying when confronted about it.

I'm still confounded by what happened, but what helps me "unstick" the trauma it created is to retell the story to anyone who will listen (or in your case, read). Whenever I do, the story always draws some laughs... and I laugh too, helping me to finally, after many years, "let it go."

Chapter 8
"Does it really take two of you to get one crummy 'B'?"

"How do you know what it's like to be stupid
if you've never been smart?"
—Lou Holtz

Leaving for college was the chance I'd been waiting for to escape the madness at home. I was anxiously looking forward to attending Michigan State, but I was also extremely upset that Stevie and I were going to be separated for the first time since we began dating…except for her New Orleans trip when she rode on "my" motorcycle. The day I was to leave, my father took me aside and said something to me that was to have a dramatic impact on my freshman year.

"Johnny, I want you to know that there is much more to learn at college than what's in the books. Do you understand what I'm saying to you?"

Is he kidding me? This is Dad saying this? Telling me he doesn't expect me to spend all of my time and efforts on studying?

"Uh, okay. I got it, Dad. I'll make sure I remember that."

Boy, did I ever! I spent so much time my freshman year learning what *wasn't* in the books that there were whole weeks I forgot there even *were* books! And I didn't intend to skip as many classes as I did, but this was cold, freezing Michigan! When the wind chill is double digits below zero, snow is piling up outside your dorm, and your first class is at eight o'clock in the morning, it's pretty easy to roll over and go back to sleep. And if you missed class, you missed class. In high school, if you skipped a day or two of classes, you could always call a buddy and find out what happened, borrow his notes (well, my friends didn't take notes, but other kids did), and get your assignments. But at Michigan State, where some lectures were attended by as many as 500 students—none of whom you knew—it was pretty tough to keep up if you chilled out (pun intended). After a while you might have met some kids in your class, but usually the people I was attracted to didn't go to class either! So it wasn't very surprising that when winter vacation began in late December, my grade point average was a tepid 2.46 (C+).

I was pretty excited to get home (well, back to St. Louis anyway) at the end of my freshman year because Stevie's break was at the same time, and we could see each other without having to spend a fortune to do so. As far as my parents, I couldn't have cared less about being in their company again. I knew that spending a couple of weeks with them would be extremely stressful and confrontational. In fact, when my father picked me up at the airport, it took less than ten minutes together in the car before he looked at me and said; "I want those sideburns off your face by dinner time tonight."

Now, you need to understand that, back in 1967, about 125 percent of all Caucasian men in college grew sideburns down to or past their ears. Many weren't just straight down, but jutted out like the sides of an isosceles triangle, with the tips almost touching the lips. To be honest, I wouldn't have blamed my father for going berserk if I had grown *those* kind of burns, but mine were fairly short (just reaching the middle of the ears), straight, and very neatly trimmed. I looked more like a kid out of the '50s than the '60s, but those sideburns still had to come off! I asked my father why, what the big deal was, and I got his typical response. "Because I said so. You live under my roof; I pay for your college, your clothes, your food, and your trips to and from school. You got any other stupid questions?"

"No, sir!" was my Pavlovian response (he had trained me well over the previous eighteen years).

Big brother Steve arrived home from his frolicking at Tulane a few days after me, without sideburns. He'd done me one better: he had a full-grown beard! He walked into the house and, in his usual fashion, flashed a couple of fingers at me to acknowledge that I was alive, and proceeded to his room, his normal spot. I couldn't help but wonder what had transpired in the car while Dad was driving *him* home from the airport. Maybe the old man told him to go straight to his room and grab his razor. Or maybe Steve headed there to find something to clobber him with. I didn't dare ask my father about the beard, so I just waited until Steve resurfaced, which didn't happen often. (I figured he would eventually have to come out of his cave to go back to the airport, if nothing else). When Steve did appear for dinner that night, the beard was still there. I spent the better part of the meal looking at Steve, then my father, then Steve again, trying to figure out what was happening. Either the old man had said something and Steve had told him to take a hike (probably not in those words) or Steve was given a deadline to meet before the ax came down. Neither of them was giving any hints, so I just ate my meal and tried to not rub my face where my sideburns had recently resided. In truth, I was pulling for Steve, figuring that if he got to keep his beard I would have a great argument for being allowed to grow back my burns.

The next day Steve actually spoke to me, but just to say that he was taking the family car to run some errands and that I'd have to ride one of our little brothers' tricycles if I wanted to go any place. Before I could protest (which wouldn't have done any good), he shocked me by asking if I wanted to go with him. That may not sound like a big deal—a couple of brothers bumming around together—but here I was, eighteen years old, and Steve had never asked me to mess around with him. I was so dumbstruck and excited that it totally escaped me that this act of fraternity never just "happened" with Steve; there had to be a catch that would result in my losing something (like money, as in the case of the motorcycle the previous year). Well, whatever he was after would have to wait: I was going to spend the afternoon with my big brother!

We were gone about three hours and I doubt we talked to each other for more than a total of ten minutes the entire time. Whenever I tried to start a conversation, I'd get a short, matter-of-fact, why-are-you-bothering-me type response.

"Hey, Steve, how's school going? I guess you're having a ball in New Orleans."

"Yeah."

"I bet your fraternity must have some great parties. You ever have them at some place in the French Quarter?"

"No."

"Really? I would have thought you would have. How's the weather been? Man, is it cold in Michigan."

"Nobody said you had to go to the North Pole to go to college. Even *you* could have gotten in someplace warmer. Hell, even Iowa would have been warmer, you idiot."

That was the longest response I got all afternoon. Maybe I hadn't missed that much by not hanging out with Steve all these years.

When we returned home, we knew something funny was up as soon as we stepped in the back door.

"Oh, boys! Is that you?"

The voice coming from the family room was friendly, almost welcoming!

"Oh boys! Come on in and have a seat!"

Steve and I looked at each other, confused and a little leery. Steve was the first to speak.

"Johnny, who the hell is that? Is that the old man? Is he on something? Has he been smoking joints? Something's up. What the hell did you do now?"

"Me? You're the one with the beard. And you're the one who looks like a Wise, not a Shuchart. *You're* the one he hates, not *me!*"

"Oh, boys! What's taking you? Come on in and sit down, I've got something I want to show you."

We made our way through the kitchen and cautiously entered the family room. Dad was sitting on his area at the end of the couch (in our dysfunctional family, everyone was assigned their own reserved part of the couch), his reading glasses resting on the edge of his nose à la Benjamin Franklin.

He was holding in front of him what looked like a couple of letters.

"Sit down, boys," he said in that same bizarre, singsong voice we had heard when we first entered the house. "Relax for a minute. Hey, I hope you guys had some fun today. You don't usually bum around together." Looking down at the papers in his hand, he said with a grin on his face, "Well now, it's kind of a coincidence how both of your report cards for the semester came at the same time, don't you think?"

We were still standing, motionless. I glanced at Steve, hoping for a hint as to what he thought was coming, but he didn't look at me. So I took a seat opposite my father. Steve sat down to the old man's right, almost out of his range of vision, leaving me to take the onslaught by myself, as usual.

The old man stared again at the papers he was holding. Then, peering over his glasses, and looking straight at me half-excitedly said, with a somewhat smaller grin on his face than he had when he first greeted us, "2.9."

"2.9?" I jumped up from my chair and screamed, "I *told* you I aced my finals. I told you I did great! *Wow!* And everyone said I wouldn't make it in college! 2.9! Baby, baby! I am the greatest!"

"Yep, 2.9," Dad replied, now quickly losing his grin along with his relatively good humor. "*TO ... GETH ... ER* you got a 2.9," his voice rising with every syllable. "And *you*, Johnny the great, got a 1.4! Now, I'd ask you to tell me what your brother over here got, but since you got a 1.4, I'm sure you're not smart enough to figure it out, so I'll help you. *Your brother beat you...* He got a 1.5!"

My first impulse was to burst out laughing. I mean, are you kidding me? Steve got a 1.5 and *still* finished ahead of me? I'm thinking we must have set some sort of stupidity record! Seriously, have two brothers *ever* combined for such a low grade point average? Fortunately I stopped myself, and Dad apparently didn't see that my eyes were about to pop out from holding back. Had I not been able to control myself, I'd probably be dead right now. I had seen my father angry before, but I could tell the next few minutes would be as explosive as any I'd ever experienced with him.

I looked over at Steve one more time. His expression hadn't changed since he'd sat down. It was like all of this was going right over his head. I was starting to sweat bullets, thinking about how I would have to go back to Michigan, pack up my stuff, come home, and enroll in a trade school, and Steve was acting like he was simply wondering what to mix with his next Jack Daniels.

My eyes left Steve and fell upon Dad just as he began to really unload.

"I have spent over 6,000 dollars this year alone so you two morons could go to schools almost geographically opposite of each other"—I have always wondered what the heck that had to do with how stupid we were—"and totally screw off!" He was now screaming so loudly that I thought his head was going to explode right then and there. "I have spent all this damn money, and I couldn't even get a B average between you un-grateful, spoiled brats! If you think for one second I'm sending you guys back so you can drink and party or whatever it is you're doing, you better think again, misters. Now, I want to know, and I want to know right *now*, just what the hell you guys think you're trying to pull. You first, Mister 1.4. Tell me just how somebody can possibly get a 1.4. You must have really worked your butt off to screw up that badly. Come on, tell me!"

By this time I was looking at my feet, scared to look at the old man. If murder had been permitted, this is the moment he would have committed it. He would have grabbed me by the neck and choked me like I was that chicken he had told me I was going to be when I was having my appendix removed. I glanced at Steve yet again, hoping to get a clue on what to do next, but I got bupkis—nothing, nada, zilch. He was sitting with his arms crossed, gently stroking his beard with his right hand. His eyes were kind of glazed over, and he was staring ahead like you do when you're totally relaxed and thinking about sex or something. I took a deep breath and, for the umpteenth time in my life, proceeded to bury myself further.

"Well, remember the day I left for school and you told me you had something you wanted to say to me? And you told me that there was more to learn than what was in the books?"

The old man, still standing, was in no mood to be asked questions. He wanted answers and he wanted them *now*!

"*Shut up!* I didn't say not to go to class, *not* to study, *not* to at least *pretend* you cared about getting an education! What I said was to keep your eyes open, to experience different things. It seems to me you haven't experienced anything new at all. You screwed around in high school and you're screwing around now! The more I think about it, the more it seems to me that your 1.4 was a miracle. I think that's about the high end of your scale (he had obviously forgotten about my insanely high, in comparison, 2.46 average the first semester, and I wasn't about to remind him of it at this particular juncture!).

"Uh, Dad, I'm really sorry. I don't know what happened. I really thought I did pretty well on my finals. I don't have a clue what happened. And as far as those three 1.0 grades, frankly, I didn't really get into those subjects. But, hey! Look at Humanities—a 2.5!"

"Your professor must have graded on the curve and 2.5 was his bottom."

I knew at that point that the more I spoke, the angrier the old man would get, so I decided to surrender. "I don't know what to tell you, Dad. It was a rough year. I know I can do better. I know I *will* do better."

"Damn right! You can't do worse!"

I kept waiting for him to turn on Steve, but he never did. I think he had long ago given up on him. Plus, Dad screaming and making threats didn't affect Steve like it did me. Steve didn't respond to intimidation. In fact, I'm not sure *what* he responded to. He kind of danced to the beat of his own drummer. Dad got much more out of hammering me than he did Steve or anyone else (including my mother). He often needed to vent his frustrations, and I was usually the one he took them out on. I'd like to say that I eventually got used to it, but I was never able to be like Steve and just let it all roll off me. Ever since I can remember, I've hated being yelled at and nothing has changed even today, regardless of who is doing the screaming.

The old man ranted and raved for another five or ten minutes, cussing and swearing about how stupid and ungrateful we were for everything he had ever done for us, especially for spending all that money to send us to college. I was pretty upset—not just because Dad was angry but because, when I thought about it, I knew I'd screwed around all semester. I hadn't gone to class very often and hardly ever studied. Now, that doesn't mean I didn't do *anything*. I did a lot . . . of drinking and staying up late and all. I knew I had let my Dad down, but what bothered me the most was that I was proving my old English teacher right; I was going to flunk out of school if something didn't change. Once I started to think about things that way, I got angry with myself and decided that I would show everybody that my second year at Michigan State would be different.

It was. Stevie was there, having transferred, and she laid down the law. We had to study every night, Sunday through Thursday, from 7:00 p.m. to 11:30 p.m. After we completed our studies each night, Stevie would give me the choice to either go get something to eat…or do something else. I won't share with you what the "something else" was, but I *will* tell you that my grades skyrocketed while my weight dropped like a rock!

Reframing a 1.4 Grade Point Average

I think you've already gathered that I knew I had screwed up. I understood why my dad went berserk and, frankly, if he hadn't, I might never have gotten my act together. Sometimes we all need a good kick in the fanny, and he had no qualms about giving me one.

It might appear that Steve got away with a lot, but I'm not sure that's so. Yeah, he got to keep his beard, and he didn't have to feel the full impact of the old man's rage, but I think Steve knew that he escaped because our father really didn't care enough about him. That had to have hurt him. Dad saw Steve as a lost cause, and short of pulling him out of school (something Dad would never have done since we're Jewish, and it's an unwritten commandment that thou shalt educate your children no matter how stupid they behave), there wasn't much he could do. I got the old man's attention all the time precisely because he did care about me. Now, I'm not saying that he was right to verbally abuse me (or anyone, for that matter), but I've come to realize that even though my father had no clue how to parent, he *did* at times try to have feelings for me.

I have mixed emotions when I look back on this chapter. On the one hand, there is no getting around how funny it was when my father told me "2.9," and I assumed that was what my report card said, only to learn that I didn't earn a grade even half that high. And, I have to admit that it was kind of neat to come within one-tenth of a point from tying Steve's grade point average, even if it *was* a 1.5!

On the other hand, I regret I wasted a whole semester of learning. I had a great time that year and made memories that remain today, but I wish I had done better, gone to more classes, and studied harder—just to please myself, not anyone else.

Looking back though, had I gotten better grades, I wouldn't have gotten to see my father reach the point where I thought his head would explode, and regardless of the tension and drama in the room that day, it really was a pretty funny encounter. As always, it's all how you frame it, and this time the picture gets funnier every time I come up with a new frame.

Chapter 9
"Your wedding? We'd rather be in Las Vegas."

"When you reach the end of your rope, tie a knot in it and hang on."
—Franklin D. Roosevelt

I knew during my sophomore year at Michigan State that I had reached the end of my rope with my parents. It seemed like nothing I did pleased them. My grades were up; I was calling home like a good boy every Sunday evening as requested, and I came home on the holidays and during vacations, again as requested. But they never truly acknowledged me. I guess by this time I should have been used to it, but I wasn't. I never got used to the slights, the constant rejections, and I especially never coped well with the fact that as much as I got clobbered when I messed up, I was rarely praised for doing well.

But, as I said, my grades were up primarily due to Stevie's rule about studying every night during the week. My initial plan for a career was to major in Russian and then work for the CIA. But while I excelled in my language studies, I gradually concluded that ducking bullets, running cloak-and-dagger operations, and risking my life daily for 400 million Americans I didn't know (and who didn't know me) just weren't the kinds of things I'd enjoy doing for the rest of my life. I decided to switch to a major just as daring but not quite as dangerous: education. I earned a teaching certificate and felt that teaching American history to teenagers would be a worthwhile endeavor. Stevie was majoring in social work, so between the two of us we knew that money would never be a problem as long as the Democrats kept supporting food stamps and other welfare programs in which we could be participants.

Speaking of Stevie, long-term romances can be tricky, and if you count from when we first met way back in pre-kindergarten, by the beginning of our junior year in college we had known each other for sixteen years. We'd been going steady since the end of tenth grade and had gotten pinned in college. By the end of our sophomore year, there wasn't much left to do except keep dating until we tired of each other or get married and look forward to spending those food stamps. We chose the latter and got engaged during the summer before our junior year—but, of course, not without my family's usual drama.

If I'd wanted to do one thing that would kill my old man—something that would bring on the "big one"—telling him I was getting married would probably have done it. But telling him I was marrying *Stevie*? I'm surprised he survived, especially since I told him the good news while he was in the hospital recovering from a gunshot wound. It seems Dad's business partner liked money more than he liked Dad and decided to try collecting on a life insurance policy on my father's life sooner rather than later. The partner was never convicted for hiring the two thugs who botched the homicide attempt; he was put away for mail fraud instead, but there's no doubt in my mind (or anyone else's) that he had tried to have the old man knocked off.

Anyway, my father was lying in his hospital bed when I told him I was getting engaged. I didn't want to share the news with him at that point, but I'd already told my mother and she insisted he be told, regardless of his condition. (Remember, she wasn't too crazy about dear old Dad either and was probably thinking that even though a bullet couldn't kill him, we shouldn't give up trying.) As it turned out, telling him was more dangerous for me than for him, for as soon as I got the word "engaged" out, he went absolutely postal. If it weren't for the dozens of tubes attached to him I'm sure he would have jumped out of the bed and strangled the life out of me. Instead, he just lay there and screamed.

"You have got to be kidding me! I'm lying on my back with a bullet in me"—not true, they had already removed it, but I wasn't going to point that out just then—"and you're telling me you're getting married? You stupid idiot. What are you going to live on? You're still in school, remember? You think school is free? Do you and your little friend have some money saved up somewhere?" (I assumed "little friend" meant Stevie, but I'd never heard him refer to her in such a kindly manner.) "You had better, because let me tell you something: if you're old enough to get married, you're old enough to support yourself. You are cut off as of right now. Good luck, dummy! Now get out of my room. I'm through with you!"

I looked at my mother, who was shuddering in the corner of the room, and knew immediately that she was not going to be any help. She had this look on her face that said, "Well, you've really done it this time." Thanks, Mom!

The rest of that summer was as tumultuous as any I have ever spent. Dad was in the hospital for thirteen weeks, caught in a cycle of infection, recovery, infection. He finally returned home and, for two or three weeks, was a changed man. He seemed to have lost his temper and gained an appreciation for the support his family had given him. My mother had slept for weeks at a time at the hospital. I'd showed up almost every night. Steve—well, I think his initial response when I'd called to tell him Dad had been shot said it all.

"Steve, wake up." (It was 4:30 in the morning.) "It's Johnny."

"Johnny? What...what do you want? This better be important, kid."

"Steve, Dad's been shot! He's in the hospital. You need to come over."

"Really? What time are visiting hours?"

That's Steve for you, especially when it came to our father. Turns out he did show up...*during* visiting hours! In fairness, by now Steve was married and finally out of our parents' reach, and as long as Dad's shooting didn't directly, imme-diately affect him, there was no way he was going to do anything to inconvenience himself.

But Dad's transformation didn't last long. A few weeks after coming home, his business faltered, something his partner knew was going to happen—thus the need to cash in on the life insurance policy. Overnight we went from being rich to being poor. My father had sunk everything into his finance business—heck, even money I'd been given by relatives had been scooped up and invested (always without my knowledge, of course)—so we lost everything. My parents sold their house in days, losing a great appreciating asset, and rented an apartment not far away.

"Johnny, it's only temporary. We'll be back in a nice home soon," Mom told me, somewhat unconvincingly. This "temporary" arrangement lasted over thirty years; my parents were never again able to afford another house.

Taking a page from Steve's book, I decided that I had a life to live and that I was moving forward with it. I was going to get married the following summer, and that was just the way it was going to be. I would work through the current summer in a construction job, saving up as much money as possible since I knew that "if you're old enough to get married, you're old enough to support yourself." After all, between college tuition and other expenses, Stevie and I would need as much cash as possible.

That fall, she and I returned to school, not knowing what— if anything—my parents would be contributing toward my tuition and living expenses. Stevie's parents continued to fund what turned out to be her final year (she graduated in three years so she could plan our wedding and support us through my senior year). After all, Stevie's parents *liked* her! And though they weren't too crazy about my folks, they accepted *me* 100 percent and always treated me with great love and kindness. I was definitely going to be the son they never had, warts and all. They supported our decision to marry, and even though I'm sure they wished we had waited a few years, they were excited to host a nice wedding for their eldest daughter.

To my surprise, my folks came through, at least for my junior year. They decided to continue to pay for my college and living expenses. They even let me keep one of their cars at school. It wasn't until several months into the school year that their support came to screeching halt.

I can't remember what triggered it for me, but early that winter I wrote Mom and Dad a "dear parents" letter (sort of like a "dear John" letter). I told them I was fed up with being treated like a loser and was sick of their constant harassment and verbal abuse. I recapped the previous twenty years of pain they had inflicted upon me, and then I hit the hot button: money. I dared them to take back their car and stop supporting me. I told them that the only thing in the world they held over me now was money and that they could take theirs (the little they had left) and shove it. Give me nothing, get nothing became my mantra and a fair exchange.

I sent off the letter and didn't think much about it. A few weeks later, there was a knock at my apartment door.

Standing there was my dear brother Steve and his wife.

"Yikes! What are *you* doing here?"

"Hi, kid," he said matter of factly. "Let's go to dinner. Call Stevie."

"Dinner? Why are you here?" I said as I let them in and they grabbed a seat on my decrepit Salvation Army couch. "You wanna tell me what this is all about?"

"Well, kid, you said you wanted the old man to take back your car, so that's why we're here—to drive it back home."

"*What*? You're doing Dad's dirty work? After all I've done for you, all the times I've taken a bullet for you? The money

I've given you that you've never paid back? The times I've lied for you? Helped you in and out of the house after curfew? And the motorcycle fiasco! Are you kidding me?"

I was beyond furious. My first instinct was to throw them out but, hey, I'm a poor college student and they're telling me we're going out to a free dinner. For once in my life I took the high road (sort of) and, after a few enormous breaths, told them I'd call Stevie.

We went to dinner. Stevie, as always, was gracious, although she was also appalled by what Steve was doing since she knew firsthand of the many scrapes I'd helped him out of. After dinner, Steve and his wife dropped us off at my apartment and that was that: Sayonara, car!

I was determined to bounce back, to show my parents that their money couldn't affect me. So the next day I went looking for a car. I had about 600 dollars to my name and I found a 1963 Dodge Dart for 610 dollars. Stevie gave me 25 dollars (the car would need gas), and within a couple of days I had some wheels again. Never mind that the car was a piece of junk, had no air conditioning (most cars back then didn't, but mine—er, now *Steve's* car—had), and would last me about six months before it fell apart, but I had taken my parents' best shot and survived!

By the time summer rolled around and plans for the wedding were in full steam, I had started talking with my parents again. My mother had called me and acted like nothing had happened, even asking me how I liked my new car (you never knew what that woman would do next, and her calling *me* was certainly a surprise). One thing led to another, and when I came home that summer, I found myself living in their apartment. My father wasn't saying much, which was, of course, nothing surprising, but my mother actually treated me in a much different way. She knew she couldn't control me with money and that I was getting married in a few weeks, so I think she decided that since I would soon be Stevie's problem, she had better begin to let go. She was very pleasant and almost supportive whenever we talked, except on one subject: the wedding.

If ever a positive event like a wedding could implode an entire family, this was the event, and mine was the family. Due to a series of misadventures, my parents created enough friction between us to make me move out of their apartment and into Stevie's parents' basement for the ten days or so leading up to our wedding. Most of their anger centered on the fact that I was getting married, period, but they used the details of the planned ceremony to try to excuse themselves from attending. And they succeeded. A few days before the wedding, they left for Las Vegas. (This, by the way, was the first "vacation" they had taken in more than twenty years, and it was to be their last.) We all assumed they would be a no-show the day of the wedding, but just as the procession began, they appeared. They refused to walk me down the aisle or participate in any way, other than to sit in the audience and embarrass themselves. After the ceremony they vanished, making sure they could always maintain they *attended* my wedding but that they in no way *celebrated* it.

They were the losers. I gave the best speech of my life at the reception, never once referring to then, but making sure everyone present knew how grateful I was for their support and understanding. My brother Steve and his wife stuck around for most of the dinner, but were the first to leave the gathering by at least two hours. Figured.

Reframing "I Do" When My Parents Said, "We Don't!"

I can't resist stating that this slight from my parents on my wedding day really took the cake. I guess I can think of reasons (none valid, mind you) why parents might choose to intentionally miss their son's wedding, like his marrying outside his race or religion, or marrying outside of his social class (assuming that's a big deal to the super wealthy), or if he were expecting to be a father sometime during the next few months and that was a deal killer. But none of these applied to me; I was just marrying a very nice, bright, beautiful young Jewish lady.

If you think I eagerly reached out to my parents after that, think again. After Stevie and I returned to St. Louis from our honeymoon, we stayed with her parents as we packed to go back to East Lansing for my final year of college and the start of Stevie's new job as a social worker. I never once spoke with my parents during that time. They didn't call me (and they knew we had returned home) and I didn't call them. I still wasn't speaking to them when a few years later we had a son, Scott, and it's only because Stevie is the most incredible person ever that my parents got to see him. Stevie insisted, over my (at times) vociferous objections, that

Scott needed to have a relationship with his grandparents, regardless of how atrociously they had treated us. So we would drive up to my parents' apartment, and I would sit in the car while Scott and Stevie went in and visited.

I wish I could say that I wasn't affected by the estrangement, but I'm a sensitive person (how that happened, living in my family, is a great mystery), and every so often I would think about calling my mother to start a discussion. I figured that she, in particular, was probably upset too, and would like to do something to erase her pitiful performance at my wedding, but I just couldn't bring myself to make the call. I was so tired of being hurt that, for my own emotional safety, I stayed away.

The pain as it pertained to my wedding started to subside when I began to realize how much it was affecting me. It took time, but my ability to use humor helped me lessen my trauma. I started to feel better when I thought about the only really funny aspect of the entire fiasco: my parents running off to Las Vegas. I guess you can't appreciate just how crazy that was unless you understand how much they each disliked traveling. As I said above, they hadn't had a vacation with just the two of them in twenty years! They occasionally took my younger brothers to a few places, but never left by themselves...ever! Now, their son was getting married and they suddenly had a burning desire to skip off to

Vegas? My mother hated crowds, gambling, and eating (she was anorexic for much of her adult life); and my father played poker only occasionally just to get out of the house and away from the craziness that was her. There were no two people in the world less likely to enjoy a weekend in Las Vegas. I'm telling you, the odds of them skipping my wedding were probably one in 10 trillion (I never thought my mother would be able to live with herself), but the odds of them going to *Vegas* instead were—well, there were no odds.

As soon as I could appreciate how hilarious my parents' escape was, I felt some relief. It felt good to think about this traumatic time in my life and be able to laugh, even just for a few seconds, because those moments allowed me to associate more relaxed, comfortable emotions with what had happened. Instead of tensing up and feeling stress from those memories, I was now able to smile and release a few endorphins.

Years later when I finally decided to contact my mother, she was excited to hear from me. The silence had been broken. But unfortunately, the drama with my Dad was about to kick into an even higher gear.

Chapter 10
"Johnny, Dad screwed it up again. The man just can't kill himself!"

"The great thing about suicide is that it's not one of those things you have to do now or you lose your chance. I mean, you can always do it later."
—Harvey Fierstein

It took less than a week for me to determine I had made a huge mistake in rekindling any kind of relationship with my parents. Mom and Dad invited Stevie and me to dinner at their place, along with my wonderful grandparents, the Wises. We walked in the door around five thirty that night, knowing that dinner would be served at six o'clock just like it had for the past umpteen years. I wasn't surprised that we beat the old man home; he had finally started a new company selling insurance. He had an office not far from the apartment, and I knew we'd see him walk in the door at the usual time, about fifteen minutes before dinner, which would be served precisely at 6:00 p.m. as always. I sat down with my grandfather, who had already arrived, and we shared some Chivas Regal (his lunchtime and pre-dinner beverage of choice). It wasn't until six o'clock had almost arrived when my mother asked no one in particular if they had heard my father come in yet.

Grandpa and I immediately looked up at each other. Something was wrong, very wrong. The old man was never late; it was against his constitution. Gramps spoke first.

"Johnny, maybe we got lucky and he split! That no-good S.O.B...." (That sort of summed up what he thought of my father.)

"No, Grandpa. He doesn't have any money; he's not going anywhere. You think maybe he's had an accident or something?"

He just smiled and slowly held up his glass of Chivas. "L'Chaim!" he bellowed.

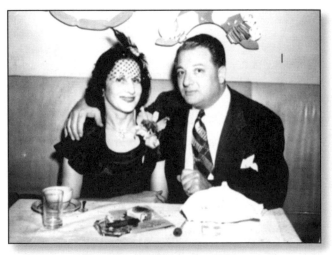

Grandma and Grandpa Wise.
They were terrific grandparents but horrible parents!

By now I figured the old man was probably lying in a ditch somewhere, and my grandfather wasn't waiting to start the celebration. I told him to get serious for a minute—that we really needed to think about this. I said that if the old man didn't show up in fifteen minutes or so, I was going to go out hunting for him. My grandfather sort of grinned, shook his head, and took a few more sips of his drink without saying anything. I have to admit, I was hoping Dad would walk in just so I could scream at him for being late just as he always did to everyone else who didn't keep his commitment to be on time: remember, this was the man who lived by the "Yes, Sir! No, Sir! No excuse, Sir!" military mantra, and I wanted to see if I could trap him into blurting out some excuse-ridden rationale for why it was okay for *him* to be tardy.

I never got the chance. The old man never did show. By six thirty I finally convinced Grandpa that we had a problem and needed to go out on the prowl. He gulped down the rest of his Chivas, grabbed his coat, and, grumbling all the way, followed me out to the car. As I started the engine, it dawned on me that I had no clue where I was going. I looked at Gramps and he just shook his head a couple of times. Neither of us knew how to find someone who was never late, never lost.

"Grandpa, what do you think? Should we hit some bars? Maybe he's out drinking or something."

"Johnny, I'm thinking he's at his office. Now, I don't have any idea why he'd be there, but this guy has no friends and no place to go. So he's either dead someplace or he's sitting in his office doing whatever he's doing. Let's go there. I don't want to ride around all night looking for him anyway. He's either at his office or he's no place—that's the way I figure it."

"Gramps, there's no way he's at his office. He's in trouble or he'd be home. We need to ride around and see if we can find him."

So, that's what we did. After about two hours of looking in bars and restaurants and finding nothing, Gramps told me to either go to my father's office or go home and start the partying.

When we got to the office we could see lights on inside, but the door was locked. My grandfather told me to go find the building supervisor and have him let us in. As soon as we got the door open, we could see my father's foot on the floor, under his desk. We walked in and there he was, passed out cold, one shoe off, one shoe on, and a half-empty bottle of Jack Daniel's Black on the desk along with an opened bottle of aspirin. We called 911 and had him whisked off to the nearest hospital. As luck would have it, the Intern on duty that night turned out to be an old high school classmate of mine. When I asked him how serious things were, he smiled and assured me that the old man had consumed just enough aspirin to relieve a headache and just enough bourbon to knock him out for a couple of hours.

I was pissed! (And Grandpa was extremely disappointed that it wasn't more serious.) What a "stunt"—Dad's favorite word after "stupid"—to pull on us! I told the Intern that if there were anything he could do to help my father feel some pain I would fully support him. He said it certainly wasn't out of the question in situations like this to pump the patient's stomach, just in case he'd swallowed something other than what was in the aspirin bottle. I was all in! My buddy smiled and said he'd get right on it. The old man might have ruined my dinner, but he wasn't going to forget doing it anytime soon.

I didn't find out until the next day what was really going on with him. It turns out he'd fallen into even more financial difficulties and had decided the only way out was to kill himself—or, in this case, to dupe us into thinking he was trying to kill himself in hopes he'd gain sympathy from somebody who might bail him out.

Despite everything I knew about my dad, I concluded that he was my father for better or worse and that dying over money didn't make much sense. The amount he owed well exceeded my capabilities, so I had to seek out the two people in the world that disliked him the most: Grandpa Wise and my Uncle Mike, whom my father had screwed over in a former business partnership. Neither was real happy when I asked for their help, but they both understood that Dad was my father, and they felt I deserved the opportunity to help him. I'll never forget the advice that came with my Uncle Mike's check, however.

"Johnny, you need to have the chance to help him…once. And I'm telling you now, you will never get your money back—*and* this won't be the only time he'll come knocking on your door. Helping him once is like walking in the winning run in the bottom of the ninth to him; he'll assume you're a wild-ass pitcher who will do it again and again. So, I'm going to help you help him this once, but don't come to me or your grandfather ever again; and if you're smart, you'll realize the next time this happens that you already helped him once, and that once is enough."

Wow…what an amazing uncle. He gave me the chance to be able to live with myself—to not turn my father away, to help him when he most needed it. But he also helped me to understand that once was enough and that I would need the courage to walk away when it happened again.

Uncle Mike was right on. It did happen again. And, yet again. Three times my father "attempted" to commit suicide, and each time it was because he needed money. Thanks to Uncle Mike's words of wisdom, which I was to adopt as my own, I turned my father down each subsequent time. And, of course, he didn't die either time, living on for many more years even after his final suicide threat.

Reframing Dad's Suicide Attempts

Anyone who has had a family member commit suicide knows how difficult it is to fend off deep feelings of guilt, whether warranted or not—even though they are rarely, if ever, warranted. But you still always wonder what you did, what you should have done, and what you could have done to prevent it. Thus, I was furious with my father for threatening something as devastating as suicide in order to manipulate his family into doing what he wanted.

Dad's second suicide threat affected me the most. By that time, Stevie and I were living in Kansas City, with my parents still in St. Louis. Dad called me late one night and said he was flying into Kansas City early the next morning and that I was to meet him at the airport. Then he hung up. I remember turning to Stevie with a look of bewilderment on my face, wondering what was possibly going on. Was he ill? Was he dying? Why was he coming and why wouldn't he just tell me about it instead of hanging up and leaving me to wait and ponder?

I met him at the airport the next morning, as he requested. As he got off the plane he said gruffly, "Let's go get coffee; my plane leaves again in an hour." That was it. We walked briskly but silently down the corridor to a coffee shop and sat down. He ordered his coffee (I ordered nothing) and still didn't speak to me until his drink came. He thanked the waitress, calmly looked at me, and said he needed money, and he needed it now! He said if I didn't give it to him, he would kill himself.

"Dad, eh…we're building a new house. In fact, they dug the hole yesterday. If I bail you out again, I won't have enough money to do the house."

He didn't flinch or hesitate for a second.

"So. Then you won't build the house. I need the money. Call me tomorrow and tell me when I can expect it."

With that, he took a sip from his cup, got up, and said he had to catch his plane.

"Make sure you call me by tomorrow. Remember what I told you I'd do if you don't come through. Bye."

I sat at that table in the coffee shop for the longest time. I recalled every word my Uncle Mike had told me. If I'd ever doubted him, I sure didn't any longer. My old man was everything he had told me and more. I kept asking myself, "What sort of father lays that kind of guilt on his son…'do this or that or I'll end my life?' I mean, how do you do that to someone, anyone—but especially to your own son?"

I finally got up and returned to my car where I sat some more, trying my best to process what had happened. I knew I was going to need some help with this one, so I called Stevie, who immediately told me to call a therapist she knew. I got the guy on my cell phone and must have sounded pretty distressed, because an hour later I was in his office trying to cope. It took more than two hours, but he finally helped me understand that all of this was my father's problem, not mine. The only answer I could possibly give my dad was "no." The therapist told me he didn't see the name "Savior" stamped anywhere on my clothes and that unless he did, it wasn't my job to keep another person alive. Though there was obviously the risk that the old man would actually follow through with his threat, the therapist told me I'd have to learn to live with that when and if it actually happened (even though he told me to bet my new house that this was just another idle threat). Still, choosing to say "no" was one of the scariest decisions of my life.

How have I handled this? Well, I *didn't* handle it very well at first, but over time I've come to grips with what the therapist told me: this was my father's problem, not mine. Dad had tried to make it mine, but the only way for me to work through it was to make sure it stayed his.

I don't try to find any humor in what my father did or the horrible position he put me in, but I did get some laughs being with my grandfather that night we drove all over St. Louis, half-hoping we wouldn't find my father. Gramps was a pretty funny guy, and that evening he'd been at his comedic best trying to keep me focused and calm. He'd sensed I was afraid of what we might find, and, although I know in my heart he really didn't wish my father any serious harm, he kept me entertained and relaxed with many hilarious scenarios of what could have happened to the old man. As I deal with the trauma of my father telling me I was responsible for whether he lived or died, I can at least crack a smile or two as I picture that night with my grandfather. And, as we've seen, just such a smile helps break the relentless cycle of negative thoughts that can accompany trauma.

Thanks, Gramps!

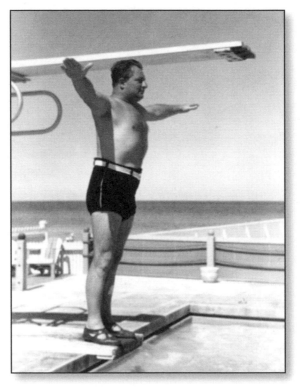

I obviously get my sense of humor from Grandpa Wise!

Chapter 11
A huge mistake with Dad; a bigger tragedy with Steve

"Learn from yesterday, live for today, hope for tomorrow."
—Albert Einstein

If there's one thing I got from my father it was plenty of advice as to the lessons I *should* have learned from yesterday. According to him, I made a lot of mistakes, which, if I had learned from them, would have given me a heck of lot of hope for tomorrow!

One of my biggest mistakes, and one that many sons make, was going into business with the old man. I had just finished up my first year of teaching school (something I was really good at and really loved) when Dad asked me to work for him during summer vacation to help him build his new insurance agency. Now, if there were two things in the world I didn't want to do, ever, they were to sell insurance and to do anything on a daily basis with my father. I ended up doing both.

My insurance career, like almost everything else in my life, started out simply but turned into something I could have never imagined. Just a few weeks into it, I was sitting before a gentleman and trying to sell him life insurance, arguably the most difficult product known to salesmen to try to sell. Nobody wants life insurance; nobody wants to pay for it, it never benefits the insured (he's dead when it pays out), and yet nobody ever buys enough of it (widows never think they've been left too much!). Nevertheless, I was sitting in this man's home doing my best to persuade him that he needed this wonderful product more than he needed a new stereo or television or whatever, and all during my presentation his five-year-old son was sitting on my lap. He was a really neat kid. He was smart, funny, and extremely well behaved. Well, by some miracle I actually closed the deal; the man said he'd buy some life insurance. But as soon as we completed the application he asked me a question that almost knocked me out of my seat.

"Now that we've gotten that out of the way, how about getting some life insurance on my son? Do you think we can do that?"

I couldn't believe he was actually *asking* to buy life insurance. Nobody ever *asks* to buy life insurance! At first I didn't know what to say, but thinking I should act cool, like this sort of thing happened all the time, I quickly told him that I thought that would probably be a good idea, that maybe we should go ahead and get him some. I took out another insurance application (acting as confidently as possible) and began filling it out. I was almost at the end when I asked him if his son had any nervous or mental disorders. I was already checking the "no" box when he stopped me.

"Ah, wait a minute. He does have a problem. He's mentally retarded" (that's the term we used back then). "He's even in a special school."

I couldn't believe it. I had spent the better part of an hour with this kid on my lap and he was great! Retarded? Was this man kidding me?

"Are you serious? He seems great! Well, I don't think it will be a problem, anyway. He's in great health. It's not like he's going to die or anything." With that I picked up my pen and continued filling out the application when he interrupted me again.

"John, how long have you been doing this—selling insurance?"

I kind of looked at my watch as if to say, "not very long, obviously." Before I could answer, he leaned forward and, very slowly, and very painfully, began to speak.

"My son has been turned down by at least twenty companies already. Nobody will insure him because of his retardation. Why do you think you can get him coverage?"

I had to confess that I didn't know, but that it didn't make sense to me that insuring someone in good health could possibly be a bad risk. I said that if we were selling *health* insurance, maybe a mental condition would be a problem (shows how little I knew). But, life insurance? I just didn't get it.

He told me he'd sign the application and that I could go ahead and send it in to the company, but that he knew I'd be calling him in a week or two to tell him his son had been rejected. I assured him I'd do whatever I could to get his application approved. As I was leaving he wished me good luck, smiled, and said he was looking forward to hearing from me.

I got back to the office and handed both of the applications to my father. When he looked at the first one he was pretty impressed; when he saw the second one, he exploded.

"You idiot! What's wrong with you? How stupid can you be? We can't turn in this application on a retarded kid. The insurance company will cancel our contract!" And with that, he ripped it up, threw it across the room, and stormed out of the office. I was really upset, both at him and at the insurance industry for being so naïve. I waited until I'd calmed down some and then called my client.

"Hi, this is John. I guess you won't have to wait a couple of weeks to hear from me. We decided that we won't even bother to send your son's application into the insurance company because we know we're wasting our time; they won't insure him. I am very, very sorry. I just don't understand it."

And then he said something that changed the entire direction of my life.

"Young man…if you want to do something good for people and probably make some decent money in the process, you'll find a way of insuring these kids."

"How many are there, you think? How many retarded children are there in this country?"

"John, about 4 percent of the population is retarded. So, that's about 10 million or even more."

"Wow! And none of them can buy insurance?"

"Well, you've just seen what happened to us, and my son is in great health. I'm sure some kids aren't doing as well as he is, so they may not have much of a chance of ever being insured. But, I'm telling you, there's a whole bunch of people out there who would be very excited to talk with you if you could offer them some coverage. And I'm not talking about big policies. We just want enough insurance to cover final expenses in case something happens. I want the same coverage for him that I have on my other children, that's all."

I told him I thought it was an outrage that the insurance industry was so lame, and I wished they would realize the mistake they were making. I told him I'd call him when his own policy came in, and hung up. I sat at my desk for a long time, trying to figure out why retarded children were so uninsurable. It just didn't make sense. It seemed to me that they would be *less* of a risk than a normal kid: they wouldn't be driving cars when they were sixteen; they were probably supervised more than most children, so they wouldn't be left alone to run out in front of a car when their ball rolled out into the street, etc. If anything, it seemed that retarded kids should be paying *less* for insurance than other kids.

That evening I told Stevie what had happened. She was as incredulous and angry as I was. After all, we were twenty-two years old, raised in the '60s, and weren't used to accepting things just because "that's the way they were." We both agreed this was an issue that needed to be addressed. Stevie said I should think seriously about leaving education to spend some time trying to find an empathetic insurance company. I wasn't so sure.

"Stevie, how am I going to get this done? Insurance has been around forever and nobody has *ever* covered these kids. There must be some really compelling reasons, maybe some evidence out there that says retarded kids *don't* live as long as other kids. I don't know, but it seems to me that these insurance guys have probably thought about this before and have decided it's a bad deal for them. If they can't make money insuring something, they aren't going to do it. They couldn't care less about the social side of the equation."

Stevie wouldn't back off. She was a brilliant social worker, a liberal thinker, and totally annoyed by any and all social injustices. I had a pretty good feeling about what was coming next.

"Johnny, you *have* to do this. I don't care that it hasn't been done before; you can do it! I have no doubt you'll figure it out. And once you do, you can always go back into teaching if that's what you decide makes you happy."

"Honey, two major problems. First, we'll starve to death. You make about 500 dollars a month. I make about 550 teaching. Together we're already just barely making it each month, and if I quit and basically go out on my own for who knows how long, we may have to live on just your income and there's no way we'll be able to do that. This just isn't going to work; we can't afford to do it."

"Johnny, we can! There's nothing stopping you from staying with your Dad and selling insurance to make some money for us while you're working on finding an insurance company. Yeah, there may be some tough months, but I know you're going to do this, and when you do, we'll have plenty of money! You'll sell what, a million policies, maybe more? Didn't you tell me there are more than 10 million retarded kids who can't get insurance? Just think how many you'd sell . . . you'll have the only policy in the world! Now, isn't that worth us tightening our belts for a while?"

"Oh, boy. I don't think you understand. *Nobody* has been able to do this...ever! How am I going to do it? I love your confidence, but..."

Stevie was adamant. "I'm not worried! You'll figure it out. It's important you do this for several reasons; the money is the least of them and I know you agree. You're one of the most caring and sensitive people I know, and I'm sure what happened today really hurt you when you had to tell that father that his son was turned down. Johnny, we'll make it just fine. I'm not worried at all. Tomorrow, I want you to tell your father what you're doing, okay?"

The next morning I told my father I wanted to speak with him. He had taken on a partner, so the two of them sat down with me. I explained what I was going to do, that I was going to split my time between selling insurance and trying to find a company to issue policies on retarded children. For the umpteenth time in my life, the old man erupted at me.

"Are you crazy? Are you the retarded one? *Nobody* is going to ever insure those kids! Don't you think they would have already done so by now? Don't you think there's a reason why they don't? You think you, of all people, are going to talk some great big multi-gazillion-dollar insurance company into doing something they've never done before? No, I'm sorry, son, but you are *not* going to split your time. You are going to do what you're supposed to be doing and that's selling life insurance for this agency. You understand, mister? Am I making myself clear? Don't let me catch you wasting time on this stupid idea of yours. Now get out of here and go sell something, for God's sake!"

I ignored my father's command and *did* split my time for the next three years. Half the time I sold insurance, and half the time I went about trying to convince someone in the industry to insure the kids. Every single Friday, at exactly

5:00 p.m., I met with the old man and his partner to review my sales for the week. Each meeting began with me telling them what I was doing, and each ended with both of them screaming at me to stop screwing around with this crazy, "retarded" idea. I ignored them every week and trudged on.

After contacting over 300 insurance companies—writing, calling, traveling for visits, and spending every dime Stevie and I had—I finally hit pay dirt and convinced a company to take a gamble on these kids. Somehow, news of what I'd done got out, and the press in St. Louis swarmed all over the story. I had a full-page feature article in the newspaper and was on the television and radio. Everyone wanted to know how I'd done it, how I'd persevered, and so on. Everybody, that is, except my father and his partner. The big newspaper article hit over a weekend and when I walked into the office Monday morning, the two of them were waiting for me.

"Well, Mr. Shuchart," my dad greeted me, holding up a copy of the newspaper. "What a great article! Congratulations."

His partner was next. "Well, it seems to me that you're going to be making a lot of money off of this, right?"

"I hope so," I said, not having a clue what he was getting at. My dad didn't keep me in the dark for long.

"Since you did all of this while you were working for us, I guess we each own a third of this thing. If you can recall, we paid for your office all this time, gave you leads for some of your life insurance sales, and provided lots of free secretarial help whenever you asked for it. So, how do you propose we set up our new corporation?"

I don't know the words for what I felt. I remember telling myself that this couldn't be happening. I mean, these were the guys who, every single Friday for three years, had screamed at me, threatened me, told me how I was wasting my life away, and ordered me to start selling more of their firm's life insurance policies (they made money on every contract I sold). And now…*now* they were telling me they owned two-thirds of my efforts? They were the crazy ones!

I sat there in my chair for what seemed like hours, but it was only a minute or so. I finally got up, looked my father in the face, and told him that I never wanted to talk to him again. I told him he was the poorest excuse for a parent ever and that him screwing his own son was absolutely beyond belief. I walked to my desk, grabbed my important papers, and walked out of that office for the final time.

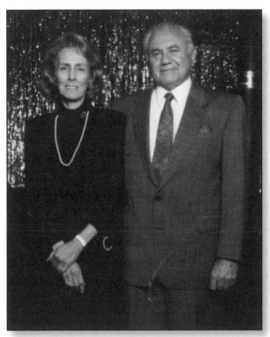

Mom and Dad acting happy…a rare occurrence!

Two important things happened over the next couple of years. First, my new company flourished. We sold policies for Exceptional Children throughout the country. (Fortunately, the "retarded" label had been dropped.) In fact, I was even contacted by parents in Canada, Mexico, and the United Kingdom. And second, I kept my word and would have never again contacted my father had it not been for what happened on April 1, 1975.

I was in my office when my secretary told me there was a phone call for me, and it was my mother. For as long as I live, I will never be able to extract from my memory the shrill I heard when I picked up the phone.

"STEVE IS DEAD! STEVE IS DEAD! HE KILLED HIMSELF!"

She hung up, and I tried to just hang on. I felt like puking. My head exploded in pain and the room started spinning. I didn't know what to do. Nothing in my life had prepared me for this, absolutely nothing. I stood up and almost fell over; my knees were wobbly and I could barely keep my balance. My secretary came in, and when I told her what had happened she started crying and had to sit down herself. I remember taking several big breaths and telling her that I was leaving and had no idea when I'd be back.

I figured my mother was at Steve's apartment, which was about six or seven miles from my office. I don't think I've ever driven so fast without looking around for cops. I didn't even think about my speed or getting stopped; all I could focus on was that Steve was dead. I almost missed the exit on the freeway and had to cut off a couple of cars to reach it. The other drivers blared their horns at me in anger. "Screw them," I remember thinking, "they don't know what just happened… they don't know I just lost my brother."

When I pulled up to the apartment, a police car and an ambulance were outside. As I got out of my car, the paramedics were rolling my brother to the ambulance. It was horrible, seeing Steve with a sheet pulled all the way up over his body. I probably would have lost it right then and there, but something told me to hold it together, that my mother needed me. I walked inside the apartment and there sat my mother, along with our foreign house sitter (don't ask, it's a long story!). Again, I had no idea what to do, what to say, so instinctively I sat down on the arm of Mom's chair and just hugged her as she wept. It was, and remains today, the most horrible moment I've ever lived through.

Steve had been having marital problems for about a year. He had a three-year-old daughter, and a divorce was the last thing he wanted, but his wife had other needs. He loved having a family, and I know that he had an extremely difficult time living alone, going through the whole dating scene, and seeing his daughter only on weekends. It wasn't the life he wanted, and so one day he decided to end it.

How I've Reframed My Father's Greed and My Brother's Death

Thanks to Stevie's incredible support, I was able to accomplish something that had never been done in the history of the insurance industry. And, thanks to my dad, I learned at a relatively young age some valuable lessons about money and the effects it could have upon the morals and ethics of some people.

Looking back, I'm proud of myself for ignoring my Dad and his partner, and for taking their verbal abuse every Friday afternoon and yet not giving in. I knew that finding the coverage for these kids was important, that it was the right path to pursue, and that even if I failed I would never look back and regret the effort I had put into it. I'd be lying if I said I wouldn't have liked my father's support but, frankly, I hadn't had much of that from him in anything I did. Living with him was a constant battle of doing it his way or "the highway."

I still don't know what possessed me to agree to join his insurance agency in the first place, unless it was a child's innate drive to be loved by his parents. And if that's why I did it, I should have known it would never happen—that my father could never, ever really love me, at least not the way I suspect most fathers love their children. I spent my entire life having him tell me how stupid I was and how I'd never amount to anything. And even when I accomplished something that many people at the time considered impossible—insuring these kids— my father never once complimented me. All he had to say was, "Where's my share?"

I've reframed this terribly traumatic episode by examining who my father really was, the kind of person who would act the way he did. I can now accept that he didn't love me—and, in fact, that he might not have loved anyone, at least not in the normal sense. In regard to the insurance issue, I had done nothing wrong; in fact, I had done everything right. I fought for something good, was able to get the task done, and in the process helped a lot of people. The loser, by a long shot, was my father. After all these years, I actually laugh when I think back to that moment when Dad and his partner told me they owned part of my efforts. The nerve of those guys! What *chutzpah*!

Steve's death, however, is a totally different matter. It's not a question of reframing what happened as much as it is trying to deal with the reality of what and why it happened. For most of us who suffer from the suicide of a loved one, the first and most harrowing thoughts we have are of whether we ourselves could have, or should have, prevented it from happening. We feel guilty; we retrace all of our steps, somehow knowing, or *hoping*, that there were signs we should have seen and therefore actions we could have taken. And that may be true in some instances, but not in Steve's case. There was nothing to be done because he wouldn't allow anyone to help him. He was a loner, secretive, very similar to my father. You never knew Steve's feelings. He was rarely "up" and never "down," at least as far as anyone could tell. Steve was, well, Steve.

In the days leading up to his death, I saw him once, and he seemed fine, just like always. In fact, thinking back, he was maybe almost better than fine—again, not really "up" but a little more talkative than normal. Normally, he didn't ask me anything about me, but this particular time he asked how my business was going, and he even asked how Stevie was doing. I've always thought that maybe his mood was a little better because he was in a good place, for him. Maybe he had already made the decision and was at peace with it.

Steve's suicide destroyed my parents as individuals and as a couple. They spent the remainder of their lives blaming each other for his death. My mother spent hours on end screaming, "Al, you killed him. You never liked him from the day he was born. I had to protect him from you every day of his life." My dad's response was equally horrible: "Jeanne, you killed him. You never let him face life. You *did* always protect him, and when he had a problem, you always jumped in the middle of it. He's dead because of you!" Living with that was almost more horrible than the actual suicide, and my parents were never able to reconcile Steve's death between the two of them. Time heals many things but not the death of a child. Ironically, my folks ended up staying together until one of them died, united more in grief and guilt than in joy.

And so, the question has to be asked . . . having lived through Steve's suicide and experienced the pain it brought to others, how could I possibly think of planning my own? For those of us who live with depression, it's more palatable. Whenever we slip into that Dark Hole of Depression, the pain and suffering exceeds all other thoughts and emotions. The feelings of hopelessness and despair far outweigh any concerns we might have for others or for how our actions may affect them. It's all about "us" when we're in the Hole. We want only one of two things: a way out, because the Hole is so horribly painful, or a way to stay in, because, ironically, sometimes the Hole is the only place we feel protected and safe.

Interestingly enough, I'm writing about Steve on what would have been his sixty-seventh birthday. I miss him, but I'm okay, and I hope he is too.

Chapter 12
"Johnny, you've been one accident after another!"

"Why fit in when you were born to stand out?"
—Dr. Seuss

I'm not saying Mom was right when she told me I'd *been* one accident after another, but I do have to acknowledge that I've *had* one accident after another! I'll start with the lawn mower.

Yes, I had a lawn mower accident. Well, I didn't have it all by myself; I had help. My son, Scott, who was about twelve at the time, was doing his typical fine job of cutting our lawn when he came into the house to tell me something was wrong with our usually reliable Sears Craftsman riding mower. The first of several ironies in this incident was that Scott actually thought I might be able to fix a broken *anything*. (I mean, we owned a "Jewish toolbox"—the kind where you open it and find the phone numbers of the electrician, plumber, and carpenter and zero actual tools.) I followed Scott outside, wondering how I would explain to him that his father had less ability in these matters than probably he himself did, and yet still retain some meaningful measure of his respect. I got lucky. It had rained the night before and the grass was damp, and some of the clippings had clogged up the blade. I pulled some grass from the blade and the mower started up just fine. No big deal, even for me.

Scott got back in the seat and resumed his mowing. I watched him for a minute to make sure everything was okay and as he drove around our swing set, the wind blew one of the swings and it got caught on the mower's clipping receptacles. As he continued accelerating forward, the swing yanked on the mower and caused it to jerk back like a horse rearing up. All I could visualize was the mower flipping over backward and crushing Scott beneath it. I yelled for him to take his foot off the accelerator but he couldn't hear me, so I ran toward him. I slipped on the wet grass and executed a slide smooth enough to gain the envy of any major leaguer, stopping just under the raised lawn mower. Scott, in a panic, jumped from the mower just as it released itself from the swing, and the 300-pound machine came straight down on my right kneecap. It bounced up into the air and landed on my gut, right next to my navel. It bounced yet again, this time aiming for my face. I threw up my arms and somehow, Jewish weakling and all, managed to flip the mower safely to the ground. Oh, I forgot to mention that the blade continued to revolve the entire time, the engine never shutting down.

I don't remember much after that until I awoke in a hospital room. Standing next to me was this gentleman dressed in a very expensive sport coat and tie, looking like he'd just stepped off the cover of GQ. He spoke first.

"Hi. I'm Dr. Hitchcock. I've been operating on you for the past couple of hours, and I'd like to ask you a question."

"Oh, really?" I think I remember asking. I was groggy and confused.

"What I'd like to know is whether you consider yourself spiritual."

Was this guy kidding? I just got run over by a lawn mower, and he wants to know if I'm spiritual?

"Uh, I don't know," I answered. "I never thought about it. Why, should I be?

"*Absolutely!* Let me tell you something. That mower didn't stop when it hit you. You have over 300 stitches in your leg, arm, and stomach. The mower's blade somehow missed every organ in your body. It's impossible that you didn't lose *something*: kidney, liver, spleen…*something!* I spent two hours doing nothing except cleaning grass out of you! Yeah, you should be spiritual…*very* spiritual."

As good a surgeon as this guy probably was, there was something he neglected to tell me. Something he'd surely noticed when he was cleaning me out. Something I didn't learn about until at least ten years later, and only discovered because of another doctor's visit. This time it was for my gallbladder. It had been acting up, so my internist scheduled me for a sonogram to see if it needed to be removed. I had the exam at a nearby hospital and was told it would take about fifteen minutes from start to finish. I was watching the clock, and after twenty-five minutes or so I asked the technician if something was wrong.

"Well, you only have one kidney, but I suspect you already knew that."

"What? One kidney? Are you serious?"

"I sure am. You mean you didn't know you had only one? Well, at least the one you've got must be working," he said, winking as he finished the procedure.

I was freaking out. I'm fifty years old and I am just now finding out I have one kidney?

"It's probably no big deal," he said. "And I see there's a pretty long scar near your navel. You must have been operated on for something, yes?"

"Yeah, I had a lawn mower fall on top of me."

"There you go! That explains it. That's probably when they took out your kidney."

"But nobody told me they took out my kidney. Don't you think they would have told me?"

"I know I would have! Maybe you should call your surgeon when we're done here. I'm sure he'll tell you all about it."

Shaken, I threw on my shirt when we finished and went to the nearest pay phone (cell phones hadn't been invented yet). I decided to call my internist first.

"Hello, Dr. Glaser? Help! I just found out I have one kidney! What do I do?"

"You've got your wallet on you, don't you?" he replied. "Take it out. Grab your driver's license. You see where it says 'Donor' on it? Scratch that out, quick!"

He started laughing, very proud of himself and his little show of humor.

"John, don't worry about it. You've got two kidneys. Many times during a sonogram, based upon the way you're lying, one kidney can sometimes be kind of on top of the other, and they can only see one of them. That's what happened, I'm sure. Relax!"

I hung up but I was still concerned, so I decided to call the surgeon—the guy who had wanted to know if I was spiritual after spending two hours cleaning grass out of my gut. I took out another quarter and dialed his office. I got his nurse.

"Hello, this John Shuchart, and I need for you to do me a favor," I told her. "Would you please look in my file and see if Dr. Hitchcock removed one of my kidneys when he operated on me a few years ago?"

She didn't miss a beat.

"Why, sure, Mr. Shuchart, I'll be happy to go check. You hold on and I'll be right back." About two minutes later she got back on the phone.

"Well, I have looked everywhere, Mr. Shuchart. In your file, around the file cabinet, in the waiting room, and I can't find your kidney anywhere!" After a perfect pause, she chirped, "Don't you think if we took out your kidney we would have told you?"

"Uh, I would have hoped so, but I just found out I only have one kidney, and it's the first I've ever heard about it. I'm trying to find out if I was born with just one or if somebody took it out sometime."

"You mean, like when you weren't looking?" And then she started laughing.

I hung up and tried to wrap my head around this development. *Okay, if I was born this way, I've lived this long—so I guess I'll continue to be just fine as long as I don't volunteer to donate a kidney. But maybe I wasn't born with just one; maybe somebody took one out. If so, who and when?*

And then it hit me. My appendicitis, when they cut me open like a chicken back when I was five years old. Did they take my kidney then? Maybe my parents asked them to take it out. Maybe they sold it on the black market! To this day I still don't know what happened to my kidney, but I'm not discounting the possibility that my parents were somehow involved!

The lawn mower accident was awful and the one-kidney discovery was weird, but they weren't life changing. That distinction was left to an incident that occurred about fifteen years ago.

I was out driving my car one day and had gotten about a mile from my house. I was making a left turn on a green arrow when an oncoming truck driver, lugging behind him some cement blocks, ran his red light and hit me at full speed. Everything around me exploded—the airbags, the windshield, the windows, as well as the walls of the car. My seatbelt was ripped from its place, and I was thrown from the driver's seat into the passenger's as my vehicle skidded 100 feet across the roadway.

I still don't know if I'm spiritual, but I do think the gods were looking out for me that day as I miraculously crawled out of the vehicle without a scratch on me. The paramedics arrived, strapped me to a board, and rushed me to the hospital. But after hours of x-rays, they found nothing. I was fine.

With two of my nine lives now used up, I was sailing along just fine until one day, a couple of years later, I felt a stabbing pain in my right shoulder. When it persisted I consulted an orthopedic surgeon, figuring I'd developed bursitis or something. As he examined my shoulder, he asked if I'd gone through any recent trauma. "Of course," I said, "I'm married!" He got a nice chuckle out of that but then turned serious.

"John, have you lifted something heavy over your shoulders lately, or thrown a heavy carry-on bag up into one of those bins on an airplane? Or have you had any major accidents?"

I thought for a second and told him that, like most people, I flew a lot and, sure, I always had a bag or two I brought onto the plane.

"And, how about an accident? Have you had one of those recently?"

"Nope. Well, I had a car accident a couple of years ago, but it was no big deal. Nothing happened to me." To my surprise, he didn't let the accident drop.

"Tell me about it," he asked. "When was it and what happened?"

I told him I was T-boned by some idiot lugging cement blocks, and so on. Then the surgeon told me to hang on, that he'd be right back. He left the room and returned a couple of minutes later holding one of those magnetic paperclip dispensers, the kind you shake and the paperclip pops up through the round opening at the top.

"I'm afraid I've got some bad news, John." He shook the paperclip dispenser back and forth a few times. "See that? That's what happened to your body when you got in the accident. Just like these paperclips, your insides have been bounced around. I hate to be the bearer of bad news, but I don't think this particular shoulder problem is the only issue you're going to be having. I think there will be more problems with your body as time goes on. If you were hit as hard as you say, then your insides got shaken like these paperclips."

I've said that my car accident was life changing, and this is why: from the date of my shoulder exam until today, I've had

fifteen surgeries to repair an issue that arguably can be attrib-
uted to the accident. Each time, what appeared to be a simple
injury to fix evolved into a complex, excruciating one. And
each time, I sank into more and more despair.

My left hand is a good example of what has happened to
me. Of my fifteen surgeries, seven have been on it alone. The
original problem, so I'm told, was typically pretty simple to
fix. It seems that when the airbags in my car exploded from
the collision, one of them hit my left wrist. In the immediate
aftermath of the accident, I did notice a tiny, pimple-sized
brown spot on my wrist, but I had absolutely no pain and no
loss of flexibility, and the mark disappeared in just a day or two.
It wasn't until a few years later that I started experiencing pain
whenever I moved my left thumb. I subsequently learned that
the De Quervain vein in my hand had been knocked out of its
channel, presumably from the force of the airbag detona-
tion. Usually whenever that occurs, the patient has surgery
and the vein is put back in place, and after a few weeks of
physical therapy the hand is as good as new. Of course,
we're talking about me here, so I should have expected the
unexpected.

My doctors decided that I needed the operation and told
me it would be no big deal: I'd have some pain and it would
take about six weeks of physical therapy to get back full use of
my thumb and wrist. So I did what they told me to do. I had
the operation and attended the painful therapy sessions two
to three times a week. As I closed in on the final few days
of therapy, my therapist noticed that my thumb still wasn't
moving as well as it should and that my pain level was still
very high, too high in fact. I told her I was just a wimp and

that any pain was too much pain for me, but she didn't buy it. She suggested I return to the surgeon and have my hand re-examined. That was a mistake! Don't ever go to a surgeon, who makes his living from operating on you, and ask if you need another operation. *Duh,* of course he told me I "needed" another one! And, so, I did it all over again—getting knocked out, cut open, and then being put through several more weeks of painful therapy. And still, by the end of this second iteration, I remained in pain, and with my thumb still immobile.

At this point, I was popping a couple of painkillers (hydrocodone) to help me get through the day, but not enough to create a problem for myself. That would change by the time I had operation number five. As my physical pain persisted, my emotional pain intensified. I began to feel hopeless. Who wouldn't? After each operation, I was promised that I was "fixed." All I had to do was to be a good boy, go to therapy, and I'd be as good as new. Right!

My depression deepened to the point where I needed medication for that as well as medication for the pain. First, I was put on Wellbutrin. When that didn't help, Lexapro. Then Cymbalta. Then I tried . . . and tried, and tried several others. As the depression worsened, so did the pain and so did my reliance upon opiates. My drug of choice became Nucyenta, as many as five or six a day. I was sinking into the Dark Hole of Depression, and now I was also addicted to opiates.

My paperclip body continued to fall apart. My hip soon needed replacing. My left shoulder started hurting, and before I knew it I had endured eight orthopedic procedures in addition to those I'd had on my hand and wrist. Each surgery hurt, each one took weeks to heal from, and each one pushed me deeper into despair. *Am I ever going to get well? Am I never going to feel good again?*

I finally decided that it had just become too hard. I began to believe that I'd never feel better, and since the only thing looking me in the face was aging, which would mean just that many more years of pain and suffering, I knew something had to change. And that's when I made the decision to commit suicide.

If you've read the Preface, you know that humor helped me realize how ridiculous my suicide plans were. But even after choosing to live, I knew I wanted to do something not just to remain alive but, if possible, to thrive. My adopted Uncle Mel's son, David, told me I needed to meet with Dr. Jeanne Drisko, the head of the University of Kansas Medical Center's Integrative Medicine Department. Spurred on by Stevie and my absolutely incredible therapist, Linda Moore, I met with Dr. Drisko, who, after a series of neurological and other examinations, determined that I would probably derive some benefit from neurofeedback. She said she had sent some patients to a clinic in Colorado, and they had experienced some remarkable successes. I agreed to go to Colorado for two weeks, undergo extensive treatment, and hope for positive results.

I walked into the Colorado clinic at nine in the morning and almost walked out by nine fifteen. The clinician, Jan Harr, introduced herself and told me to take a seat in front of a computer monitor. She said she'd be placing several electrodes on my head. She assured me that she was not planning to electrocute me; in fact, nothing would be entering my thick skull at all—the electrodes would be sending information about my brainwave activity to her computer. Then she asked if I'd ever played Pacman, and of course I had (hasn't everyone?). She told me that I would be playing fifteen or more rounds of the game and asked if I was ready to begin.

"Sure," I replied, with a large amount of trepidation. "I'm not sure why we're doing this but I assume you do! Where's my joystick?"

She smiled. "Well, here's the thing, John. You're going to be playing Pacman with your brain, not with a joystick."

What had I gotten myself into? I'd paid all this money (insurance didn't cover the neurofeedback or my travel expenses) and for what? This had to be a sham; how was I going to manipulate anything with my brain? I almost got up and left, but decided I should at least see what was going to happen next. So, I remained in my seat as Jan explained the deal.

"You are going to focus as hard as you can on the Pacman as he eats up the dots," said Jan. "Just focus, that's all you need to do. While you're focusing, I'm reading the information being transmitted to my computer from the electrodes I've placed on your head. For now, that's all you need to know. You won't feel anything, I promise. Nothing is being put into your head; I'm just reading what's going on in your brain."

I took a deep breath. Jan took her seat at her computer, which was right behind my monitor, so I couldn't see her or what she was doing. She began the game and for the next thirty minutes or more I "played" Pacman with my brain. He would speed up, slow down, turn colors, and eat dot after dot. After a while I decided that I really *was* playing the game, and that I was the one controlling his speed and direction. Turns out, Jan was the one doing the manipulating, making Pacman move based on the information she was receiving from me. The protocols she was using were telling her what was happening with my brainwaves whenever Pacman moved. If she determined the waves in a particular region of my brain were too short, she would direct Pacman's movements in such a way that would force that area of my brain to "exercise" itself, helping to change the length of the waves. The idea was that if Jan could help me change some of those brainwaves and create new pathways, I might see a decrease in certain issues and symptoms I'd been experiencing.

I spent my two weeks at the clinic undergoing different therapies every day, including the weekends. By the fourth day I was beginning to feel different, but I couldn't put my finger on it. I knew something was going on and that it was good, but I was still a little nervous. Jan asked me about my pain, and I told her I was feeling pretty much pain free. And then she asked me about my opiates, how many I was taking every day. I started to give my usual answer—about five or six—when I realized that I hadn't taken one pill since I got to Colorado! I had gotten off of some of the most addictive pills ever . . . cold turkey! Wow! I knew it had to be the therapy; there was no way I could have just quit on my own. Something was helping me in a very big way.

It's been four years since I went to Colorado and I haven't had an opiate since. I also don't have any more symptoms relating to attention deficit hyperactivity disorder (ADHD), a condition I'd been diagnosed with thirty years ago.

And, by the way, now I refuse to play Pacman with a joystick!

How I've Learned to Use Humor and Reframe Two Horrible Accidents

Can you imagine many things more horrifying than being crushed by a riding lawn mower with the blade still spinning? And then to wake up from surgery (at least you woke up!) and your surgeon, a man of science, only wants to know whether or not you are a spiritual person? Now...*that's funny*!

Or, imagine being told after fifty years that you only have one kidney, and they're not sure why? Your internist tells you to tear up your driver's license, your surgeon's nurse looks all over the office but can't find your kidney anywhere, and you wonder if your parents had the nefarious idea to make money off of your organ way back when you had an appendicitis. Now...*that's funny, too*!

How about being T-boned by a large truck lugging cement blocks? Your car explodes and yet you wind up with only a tiny mark on your wrist...or so you think until another man of science shakes a container of paperclips, saying it represents the earthquake your body went through when your car got clobbered. Now...*that's really funny*!

And how about paying a pretty penny to visit a clinic that is working with some of the newest, most advanced neurological techniques, and when you arrive they tell you you'll be playing Pacman . . . with your brain! *Now, that's really, really funny!*

Each one of these events was traumatic in its own way. Each one caused great pain, stress, or both. Yet, when viewed with a sense of humor, each is funny. Each is preposterous. Each couldn't have just happened—yet each did!

The lesson is that while events can hurt and traumatize, they can also be reframed. That's what I've been able to do successfully, because each time I retell these incidents, my audience laughs; their laughter feeds into my endorphins which, when released, help me reduce the trauma that these events caused me.

Incidentally, Stevie sold that infamous lawn mower while I was still in the hospital recovering. When my car was later totaled, I got a new one (which is more than I can say for the kidney we still can't find). And as far as video games go, all I need to play them with is my brain!

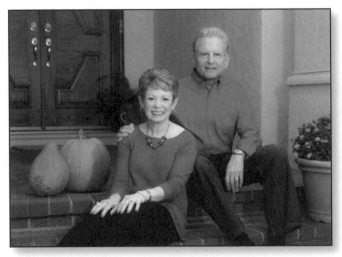

Still together and looking good!

Epilogue

Everything gets better in the end. If it's not better, it's not quite the end."
—Paulo Coelho

My life, just like yours, has been a journey with many ups and downs. Since birth I have lived with mental illnesses (ADHD and depression) that have at times been exacerbated by my environment and the people in it. I was raised in a home that many therapists would label as being verbally abusive by parents who tried to do their best at parenting, but fell short of providing the nurturing and support that I personally needed. Their rocky marriage and constant bickering, along with their own mental illness battles (especially my mother's), negatively affected my older brother Steve and me in different ways. Steve became reclusive whenever he was in our home, and although he tried to ignore what was happening, he couldn't, and never developed the coping skills that would allow him to handle his divorce and separation from his family. His premature death will haunt me forever.

In my opinion my younger brothers were probably affected too, in somewhat similar ways, but as I've discussed in the Introduction, they were raised more like grandchildren at times than children. My parents were older by the time that they had them, and after raising Steve and me, they changed from being strict disciplinarians to being much more flexible in their parenting style. However, the environment, at least from the few times I was present to observe, hadn't changed much, as the fighting and screaming seemed to continue. It's interesting to note that my brother Fred looks a lot like me, while the youngest in the family, Jay, resembles Steve. And, not surprisingly perhaps, Fred was much closer to our father than was Jay…who, like Steve, looked more like my mother and her side of the family. This was a big problem for Dad with Steve and maybe with Jay, too. I wasn't present enough to observe Jay's relationship with my father, other than on rare occasions, but those instances seemed to reveal that perhaps Dad struggled with mental illness issues that were never acknowledged and treated.

I'm almost sixty-six years old now, and I'm in a better place than I've ever been before. It hasn't been easy, but as I've tried to share with you, I've learned to manage my mental illness. The neurofeedback I undertook after my traumatic automobile accident helped eliminate any physical remnants of my ADHD (it created new pathways and increased the length of certain brainwaves), and as a result I can say that I no longer experience most of its symptoms. My legs don't have to be pumping up and down while I'm sitting, my mind doesn't wander when I am reading, and my attention span and ability to live in the moment have greatly improved.

My battle with depression, of course, isn't over. The neurofeedback I underwent no doubt improved it, but certainly didn't cure it. However, reframing the many traumatic events of my life has helped me get to this better place that I'm in. Using humor to take the sting out of a painful event works for me: it helps me to laugh, which releases those feel-good endorphins in my body, which helps keep me from sliding back into that Dark Hole of Depression.

This book, as I've stated previously, is about me and my life experiences, and how I've learned to use humor in my struggles with depression, the terrible stigma associated with mental illnesses, and words that have hurt me. It's also about helping readers to understand that those of us who are living with a mental illness are not helpless. We *can* learn to manage our illnesses, and we *can* become successful, contributing members of society. However, in order to give ourselves the best chances to thrive in society, we need to finally address the stigma that goes along with living with a mental illness.

Not long ago, *The New York Times* ran two impressive articles, one on post-traumatic stress disorder and the other on new ways some researchers are viewing mental illness as it relates to environmental factors, as well as to biological abnormalities. Shortly thereafter I saw that two different cable networks had shown pieces on mental illness and its stigma. The point is that the public is becoming interested in mental illness, what it is and what it isn't, and how we as a society need to address it. However, eliminating the stigma won't be easy. It also won't happen fully until we educate ourselves about mental illness and begin to successfully encourage those living with the disease to share their stories about their own personal struggles, and to demonstrate their abilities to capably manage their problems when proper care is made available to them.

We have made real progress in diminishing the stigma felt by cancer patients and especially HIV patients, and this is very encouraging for those of us who are battling with mental illnesses. It was not that many years ago that cancer was such a frightening word that the stigma associated with it, almost in itself, sent patients into episodes of depression. Now, when we hear about a friend who has cancer, we often times find out from that friend herself, who by telling us about the disease, is proving that the stigma attached to cancer has been greatly minimized. As for HIV, we all can remember the horror of discovering that someone had become HIV-positive. It wasn't unusual for us to treat such a person as though they had leprosy or some other terrifying, communicable disease. It wasn't until basketball star Magic Johnson shared with the world that he had contracted the virus, that people stood up and took notice. Here was one of the all-time greatest basket-ball players in the world admitting he was HIV-positive, but that it would not derail him from living his life as normally as possible, and that it would not stop him from being himself. By saying so, he was declaring that the stigma attached to HIV was totally unwarranted as far as he was concerned. Magic's "coming out" and handling his illness the way he did changed everything as far as the public's views on HIV.

A Magic Johnson would certainly help mental illness and its fight against stigma, but in lieu of someone of his stature admitting he has the disease, the same results can occur if we *each come out of the closet*. If those of us who are living with a mental illness would begin to openly admit that we have the disease, the stigma would begin to fade. You see, if I'm ashamed that I live with depression, you'll feel my negative vibes and react accordingly. On the other hand, if I don't think living with a mental illness is something to get embarrassed about, then the odds are that you won't, either. *If I understand and help you to understand that my illness is not my fault, that I didn't do anything wrong, then we both will be able to begin to doubt the validity of attaching a stigma to it.*

One of the most important steps I've taken in the past year for my recovery has been serving on the Kansas board of the National Alliance on Mental Illness (NAMI). NAMI is the largest advocacy organization for mental health issues in the country. We offer many free courses and programs for professionals, family members, and friends, as well as for those living with a mental illness. The organization is helping hundreds of thousands of us deal with the struggles associated with the disease, and by NAMI's mere existence, it contributes mightily toward the reduction of the stigma. I would encourage you to consider becoming a member of NAMI (current dues are just $35 a year), whether or not you are directly affected by mental illness, because in fact, we are all affected, whether it be by someone we care about, someone we know about, or ourselves. Each of us should want to confront the emotional, physical, and environmental aspects that make up this disease.

I have also been fortunate to play a part in a relatively new coalition here in my hometown of Kansas City, the Greater Kansas City Mental Health Coalition. Established by Jewish Family Services of Greater Kansas City, the Coalition has grown to over twenty member organizations with the stated objective to end the stigma. Their public relations campaign, which centers on the theme that "it's okay" to talk about mental illness, has been extremely effective in helping people in Kansas City to want to learn more. Check out their website, www.itsOK.us, and consider contacting them about how to start your own local coalition.

A friend asked me the other day how I was feeling about myself and about the effort I expended on the book, now that it has been completed. He also questioned if there were some other takeaways I wanted him to know about, other than what's been stated in the book.

I told him that first of all, as I've said before, I'm doing well. My mental health, like that of many of us, is fragile, and certain stresses, environmental factors, and unknown future events can trigger my slide back into the Dark Hole of Depression. However, through the use of humor and the other tools at my disposal such as those made available by organizations like NAMI and the Coalition, I've learned how to lessen the chances that it will happen.

Second, writing the book certainly took a lot of effort. I've spent six-plus hours every day on it for almost the past year, and I have to admit that I'm tired, both mentally and physically. It's been an all-consuming project, one that I have really tried my best to get right. I can't think of a sentence that hasn't been reviewed at least ten or more times, with each chapter rewritten over and over in the hopes that it was saying what I wanted to say in the way I felt it needed to be said. I am confident the book isn't perfect. There are areas that could be better, but at the end of the day, I think you now know who I am, where my passions lie, my hopes and expectations for myself and my family, and frankly more about yourself and the work we all have to do in the area of mental health.

Finally, I said to my friend that I really believe that one day with *everyone's help*, we'll learn to manage mental illness, and when we do, we'll all break into big smiles. And then we'll laugh…and it won't matter to me or to anyone else if I'm "not the brightest" of my mother's four sons.

Acknowledgments

This book would never have been written if it hadn't been for the support I've had from family and friends. In spite of the frustration and pain I know I've often caused, people have consistently rallied around me. I know that when times have been the toughest for me, like when I've slipped into that Dark Hole of Depression, it would have been very easy for them to abandon me and to tire of my moods and my sporadic behaviors, but not one of them ever did.

My family has not just witnessed my pain; they've felt much of it themselves, seeing me at times ruminate for days on end about my hopelessness and despair. My wife, Stevie, has somehow always managed to maintain a sense of calm and confidence, helping our children live with a father they often times had trouble understanding. I can't recall but a handful of occasions in our lives together that I haven't caught her smiling, optimistic, and loving me regardless of the hurt I may have caused her. She's the most beautiful person I know both inside and out, and absolutely everyone she meets feels the same way about her as I do.

My daughter, Carrie, is an incredibly strong and resilient young lady. She has all the tools: brains, savvy, great looks, and an incredible gift of communication. She is an author, entrepreneur, corporate consultant, and public speaker extraordinaire, and has also tried her hand at doing stand-up comedy. Best of all, she tells me like it is...never sugarcoating anything (whether I want to hear it or not), always pushing me to be a better person. And, if I was ever unaware of how my illness, as it progressed, was affecting my children, her request to me a few years ago was most enlightening and alarming: "I want my Daddy back!"

Scott's achievements since his youngest days are legendary: national debate champion; class valedictorian; Harvard, Oxford, and Yale Law graduate, but one of his important contributions in life as far as I'm concerned has been his support of me. He has always been the calm I've needed, never too high nor low, just caring and rational. I know my pain has troubled him at times, and in spite of his own tremendous responsibilities as a husband, breadwinner, and father, he always has time to listen, to hug, and to reassure me of his confidence and love for me.

I have had so much support from so many friends that it would be impossible for me to thank them all properly. Most people have a handful or fewer really good friends; I have many more than I have fingers and even toes, and none cares about me more than Eric Talb. I've known Eric ever since I hired him and forced him to move to Kansas City (his wife, Linda, didn't put me on her 'A' list for some time for doing so, but she's happier here than anywhere she's ever been). He has always been honest and direct with me. He calls me almost daily just to check in and to scream at me for not returning his calls. He also is my Jewish repairman (I know, an oxymoron!), fixing absolutely everything that ever goes bust in my house. Eric's good buddy and mine, Larry Zimmerman, doubles as my attorney and there's none better (I should know; due to my many business ventures, I've worked with several). Larry is one of the most nurturing people I know; he really "gets it," always showing he cares whether with words or a warm hug. His wife, Mimi, has a personality much like mine, and we get along famously. She's a therapist, too, as is Stevie, so when we all get together, sometimes it's like attending a free psychoanalytical workshop for the rest of us.

I don't want to list all of the many friends that I owe so much to for fear I'll leave someone out, but I do have to thank Jeff Marks in particular. Jeff is not only my accountant, he is also who I try to emulate. He is the kindest, most considerate man. His actions toward everyone from custodians, to waiters, to each of his very successful clients never deviate: everyone is treated with respect and gratitude. Jeff is what is called in Yiddish a mensch…a real gentleman. I am honored to be able to say that I have him as a friend of mine.

I also need to single out Mark and Diane Davidner. Mark is a most successful oncologist, and Diane is one of the warmest people one will ever meet. As busy as Mark is, he never fails to touch base with me on occasion to see how I'm doing and to answer questions I have about his car (I love his new Beemer). Diane is one of the most upbeat people I know; speaking with her is always a joy. She gets excited about my current projects and never fails to say important words of encouragement to me. The Davidners have more children, grandchildren, and friends than any couple could ever ask for, yet they have found room to allow Stevie and me to be part of their lives. As they give generously of their time, money, and efforts to improve the community, it is easy to see why they have the love and respect of so many of us who know them.

Shelly and Stevie Pessin are not only two of our longest-running friends, they were once almost our business partners.

Shelly is (as are my wife Stevie and I) originally from St. Louis, and one day we realized that, at the time, Kansas City lacked any frozen custard stores. Frozen custard was a famous St. Louis treat, shared by only a few cities (Milwaukee comes to mind), and so we decided to open our own store and expose our town to this great dessert. Since our wives share a very uncommon name (Stevie), we were going to call it, "Stevies' Frozen Custard." Due to a comedy of errors, the store never opened, and today Kansas City has as many frozen custard stores as any place in the country (argh!).

Harry Himmelstein and Pam Feingold Brooks are two long-time, wonderful supporters. Harry calls whenever he thinks it has been too long between visits to check up on me, and to also monitor the progress of my children, which he's done since they were in elementary school. He has always gotten a kick out of their achievements, sometimes even surprising me with information he's discovered about them that I haven't yet heard about! Pam is another friend who like others, really tells me like it is. She regularly checks in on me to take a pulse on my well-being—and while always encouraging and supportive, she points out actions I need to take to help myself. If I had ever asked my mother to have another child, I would have wished for Pam to be my big sister.

My other major line of support after immediate family and friends will surprise some, but it's my wife's family members. From the moment I married Stevie, I have been accepted totally by her family. I have felt loved and respected by each of her cousins and aunts and uncles even though they have forbidden me to give any more speeches at family events (it seems my humor doesn't always stay on the straight and narrow!). Everyone in the family knows about and understands the issues that I've struggled with, and yet not once has anyone ever been dismissive of me, only showing much love and understanding. The "I married a Bohm" club is the best club one could ever be a part of!

Rick Cagan and Tina Grzeskiewicz from NAMI Kansas are two extremely dedicated leaders who are working hard to help people like me manage my illness. Rick is one of the most successful and inspiring Executive Directors NAMI has, and Tina's role as President of NAMI Kansas has allowed her to use her talents to motivate others in the fight against stigma. She has become a support person for me and for everyone she touches.

The Greater Kansas City Mental Health Coalition (www.itsOK.us) was the dream of Don Goldman, Executive Director of Jewish Family Services of Greater Kansas City. Don's tireless efforts have led to a new movement in Kansas City, one to awaken the citizens to the need to end the stigma associated with mental illness. Kim Romary, the coalition's coordinator, does an incredible job serving more than twenty different coalition members, and she's out seeking more.

Would you believe that this book project wasn't my idea? The credit goes to Jim Blasingame. I've known Jim ever since his public relations agency helped me create an HMO in St. Louis. He's a brilliant marketing and public relations guy, that's for sure, but he's also a wonderful soul. It was Jim who convinced me that my life was worth sharing and that I had the ability as a storyteller to write this book. From day one Jim has been there to prop me up whenever I thought I would never be able to write (writer's block?), and those many times when my illness contributed to some of my downward spirals. He has always been able to convince me of the worthiness of not just this project, but also of myself and of others. His heart is as big as can be, and his love of people and their inner goodness helps him to be the person that he is, which is one of the best I've ever met. He's more than a friend and business partner; he's someone I aspire to be like in many ways.

My writing isn't nearly as good as my storytelling so thanks to Marianne Wasson! She's my editor (along with lots of help from Jim) and without her the book would be a hodgepodge, and you'd be as confused as I sometimes get! I met Marianne like I meet a lot of people, which is by running my big mouth. I sat next to Marianne's mother, Barbara, on a plane one day, and after three hours of my non-stop talking, when I finally allowed her to come up for air, she told me about her daughter being an editor. I needed one, and Barbara needed me to shut up so she could give me Marianne's number. I hired her during our first phone call. I can't thank her enough for her work and for her work ethic. She has been extremely responsive (even though she has a full-time job), thorough, AND she really likes and believes in the project.

My thanks also go to the entire Mallin family (especially Mel for allowing me to adopt him as my uncle), my incredible therapists, Dr. Linda Moore and Marsha Lawrence (my physical therapist par excellence), along with Dr. Jeanne Drisko, and Jan Harr. David Mallin referred me to Dr. Drisko, who with Dr. Moore's support and backing convinced me to do my neurofeedback work with Jan. Jan herself spent two full weeks with me (hard to believe she survived as well as she did), and her neurofeedback, caring, and support helped me immensely in my struggles with depression and ADHD. To this day I do not know what would have happened to me had the neuro-feedback failed. Thanks to Jan's tireless efforts in working with me, the treatments were a huge success.

Finally, a special nod to my incredible grandchildren, Oliver and Miranda. They bring a special light and joy to my life on good days and bad. I am hopeful that my renewed health may enable me to watch them grow and blossom for many years to come.

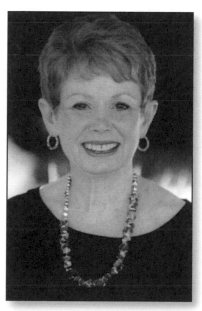

Stevie today…better than ever!

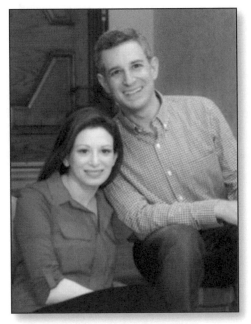

Carrie and Scott, the most incredible kids you could ever ask for!

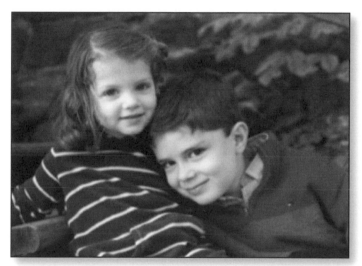

Miranda and Oliver: grandkids are the best!

About the Author

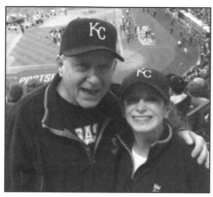

The author and his daughter Carrie, proud to
wear their Royals gear in 2014.

John Shuchart is a man of many parts. In his early 20's, he
left his middle-school teaching position and changed the
insurance industry when he made it possible for parents to
insure their mentally handicapped children. Later, he spear-
headed innovations in the delivery of employee benefits
through payroll deduction. After selling his successful insurance business, Shuchart returned to the classroom where
he worked with students to develop AFTER, a curriculum
designed to help high-school and middle-school youth work
through the anxiety caused by the September 11, 2001
terrorist attacks in New York. Shuchart led student groups
in Kansas City, New York and Israel to create their own
courses on dealing with terrorism. The program spawned
two books: *Kids' Letters to Terrorists*, and *Israeli Kids' Letters
to Terrorists*, a book for which Israeli President Shimon Peres
provided the foreword.

Referred to as a "serial entrepreneur" by the *Kansas City Business Journal*, Shuchart has created several successful businesses and worked as a marketing consultant for the past decade. He has used his business acumen to benefit a long list of nonprofit groups including: The FBI Citizens' Academy, Triality, the American Red Cross, Consensus, NAMI Kansas, Temple Bnai Jehudah, Congregation Kol Ami, Harris Youth Foundation, Greater Kansas City Mental Health Coalition, and the Kansas City Autistic Training Center. Shuchart also teaches a youth entrepreneurs program at Truman High School in Kansas City.

Throughout all of his accomplishments, John has suffered with serious episodes of depression as well as ADHD. He has proven that mental illnesses can be managed, and that those living with mental illnesses can succeed and live happy lives. With this book and his founding of The Shuchart Group, he is committed to helping put an end to the stigma associated with mental illness. A gifted storyteller, Shuchart will be entertaining organizations across the country while spreading his message of inspiration and encouragement. To contact the author about a speaking engagement, email him at john@theshuchartgroup.com or call 913-485-3336.

The Shuchart Group
P.O. Box 651
Collinsville, IL 62234
www.notthebrightest.com